MOTOR
NEURONE
DISEASE

MOTOR NEURONE DISEASE

Edited by

F Clifford Rose

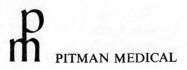 PITMAN MEDICAL

First published 1977

Pitman Medical Publishing Co Ltd
42 Camden Road, Tunbridge Wells,
Kent, TN1 2QD, England

Associated Companies

UNITED KINGDOM
Pitman Publishing Ltd, London
Focal Press Ltd, London

USA
Fearon-Pitman Publishers Inc, California

AUSTRALIA
Pitman Publishing Pty Ltd, Melbourne

CANADA
Pitman Publishing, Toronto
Copp Clark Publishing, Toronto

EAST AFRICA
Sir Isaac Pitman and Sons Ltd, Nairobi

NEW ZEALAND
Pitman Publishing NZ Ltd, Wellington

SOUTH AFRICA
Pitman Publishing Co SA (Pty) Ltd, Johannesburg

Set IBM by John Alan Graphics Limited, Tunbridge Wells. Printed by
photolithography and bound in Great Britain at The Pitman Press,
Bath, Avon.

FOREWORD

The Council of the Medical Society of London considered very carefully the various ways in which the Mansell Bequest might be used and the terms of Mrs Mansell's will fulfilled. When agreement to have a Symposium had been obtained, it was the unanimous view that the members should be the foremost national and international experts that there are representing all aspects of this field. The Society is very grateful to the distinguished workers who made time for the meeting.

It seems possible that the success of the response reflects the great need for a symposium of this kind. Although there have been great advances in knowledge of many aspects of neurology relevant to the disease, the lot of the sufferer from motor neurone disease has not improved much, if at all, in the last fifty years. This, it is thought, is what was in Mrs Mansell's mind when she left her bequest. She had watched the remorseless progress of the affliction in her husband and hoped that the Society, embodying as it does many disciplines, would direct its attention towards alleviating the lot of the sufferer.

Her bequest is not a big one. For this reason it was thought that one of the best ways of starting to use it would be to invite experts to review current knowledge and developments concerning motor neurone disease, and to point out those lines of research to which should be drawn the attention of grant giving bodies in general and of the Council, administering our own small fund in particular.

It was considered essential to publish promptly and widely the proceedings of this symposium, particularly as the numbers of those attending had to be limited. The Society is therefore glad that it has been possible to obtain the interest of Pitman Medical, who will utilise their rapid publication techniques. It is pleasant to note that in publishing this Symposium the Society will be continuing an interest in neurology which has long formed an important part of its activities. Thus among its orators are Hughlings Jackson, Wilfred Trotter, Harvey Cushing, Sir Francis Walshe, Sir Charles Symonds, Sir Russell Brain, and Macdonald Critchley.

As President, I thought it important that the symposium should be guided from the chair by a neurologist who himself is actively concerned with this field. It gave me great personal pleasure therefore that a distinguished member and ex-councillor, Dr Clifford Rose, agreed to chair the meeting and to edit the proceedings.

A W Woodruff,
President of the Medical Society of London, 1975–76

PREFACE

The first symposium on motor neurone disease was held in Paris in 1925 on the occasion of the centenary of the birth of Charcot and published in *Revue neurologique.* Further symposia were held at the Mayo Clinic in 1957 and the Royal Society of Medicine in 1962, being subsequently reported in the proceedings of these institutes. In 1967 a conference held on San Francisco on 'Motor neuron diseases' was published in 1969 (by Grune and Stratton). The last meeting on this disease, held at the Johns Hopkins Hospital in 1972, was only briefly reported (McKham, GM and Johnson, RT (1973) *Science, 180,* 221). On each of these occasions the current knowledge regarding this sad disease was reviewed, and by studying the publications it can be seen that the problems have been successively clarified and further knowledge added.

Patients with this invariably fatal disease seem all the more poignant since the intellect is preserved until the end. Not only are we still far from a cure but it is difficult to know in which field advances are most likely to come. For this reason, a multi-disciplinary approach is required and the subjects covered in this book are seen from several viewpoints: clinical, epidemiological, genetic, pathological, histopathological, clinico-pathological, virological, electrophysiological and therapeutic. It is hoped that a future symposium will include more specific remedies and this present work serve as a contribution to that end.

F Clifford Rose

CONTRIBUTORS

S Borenstein

Brain Research Unit, University of Brussels, Bd. de Waterloo 115, B 1000, Brussels, Belgium

W G Bradley
MA, BSc, DM, FRCP

Department of Experimental Neurology, University of Newcastle upon Tyne, and Deputy Director, Muscular Dystrophy Research Laboratories, Newcastle General Hospital, Newcastle upon Tyne, NE4 6BE

R C Butler
MRCP

Lecturer, Department of Experimental Pathology, Charing Cross Hospital, Fulham Palace Road, London, W6

J B Cavanagh
MD, FRCP

Director, MRC Research Group in Applied Neuro-biology, Institute of Neurology, 8–11 Queen Square, London, WC1

J E Desmedt

Brain Research Unit, University of Brussels, Bd. de Waterloo 115, B 1000, Brussels, Belgium

M Gawel
MRCP

Hon. Senior Registrar, Department of Neurology, Charing Cross Hospital, Fulham Palace Road, London, W6

J T Hughes
MD, FRCP

Department of Neuropathology, Radcliffe Infirmary, Oxford, OX2 6HE

L T Kurland
MD, DrPH

Chairman, Department of Epidemiology and Medical Statistics, Mayo Clinic, Rochester, Minnesota 55901, USA

P D Lewis
MD

Senior Lecturer in Histopathology (neuropathology) Royal Postgraduate Medical School, Hammersmith Hospital, London, W12

W B Matthews
FRCP

Department of Clinical Neurology, University of Oxford

C A Pallis
FRCP

Reader, Department of Neurology, Royal Post-graduate Medical School, Hammersmith Hospital, London, W12

Richens, A
PhD, MRCP

Reader, Department of Clinical Pharmacology,
St Bartholomew's Hospital, London, EC1A 7BE

F Clifford Rose
FRCP

Consultant Neurologist, Charing Cross Hospital,
Fulham Palace Road, London, W6. Consultant
Neurologist, Medical Ophthalmology Unit,
St Thomas' Hospital, Lambeth Palace Road,
London, SE1 7EH

J C Sloper
MD, FRCP

Director, Department of Experimental Pathology,
Charing Cross Hospital Medical School, Fulham
Palace Road, London, W6

P K Thomas
MD, DSc, FRCP

Department of Neurology, Royal Free Hospital,
London, NW3 2QG

D de B White
MB, MRCP

Registrar in Psychiatry, The Maudsley Hospital,
London, SE5 8AZ

A W Woodruff
MD, PhD, FRCP,
FRCPE, DTM and H

Director, Department of Clinical Tropical Medicine,
Hospital for Tropical Diseases, 4 St Pancras Way,
London, NW1 0PE

P O Yates
MD, FRCPath

Proctor Professor of Neuropathology, Stopford
Building, The University, Manchester, M13, 9PT

CONTENTS

CHAPTER ONE

CLINICAL ASPECTS OF MOTOR NEURONE DISEASE

F Clifford Rose

History

Before the middle of the last century, there were reports of patients who we would now recognise as revealing the manifestations of motor neurone disease (MND), notably by Sir Charles Bell, in 1830. Although Duchenne claimed priority for describing progressive muscular atrophy (PMA) in 1847, it was first called by this name by Aran in 1850. It is to Duchenne that we owe the recognition of progressive bulbar palsy, which he called glosso-labio-laryngeal paralysis, in 1860. Charcot fully delineated amyotrophic lateral sclerosis in 1865.

From the neuropathological point of view, atrophy of the anterior roots was first described by Cruveilhier in 1853 and of the anterior horn cells by Luys in 1860.

Nomenclature

The term motor neurone disease and amyotrophic lateral sclerosis (ALS) have been used interchangeably; it is preferable to restrict the latter to those cases in which upper motor neurone signs predominate, so that motor neurone disease includes in addition those cases where lower motor neurone signs are the chief feature and the term progressive muscular atrophy (PMA) is usefully applied (Table I).

TABLE I. Nomenclature of Motor Neurone Disease (MND)

1	Progressive muscular atrophy (LMN)	
2	Amyotrophic lateral sclerosis (UMN)	
3	Progressive bulbar palsy	(a) chronic (LMN)
		(b) pseudo- (UMN)

LMN = lower motor neurone   UMN = upper motor neurone

1

When the lower cranial nerves are affected, this will produce chronic bulbar palsy and, if the supranuclear innervation is affected, the features of pseudo-bulbar palsy will be present.

Incidence

The annual death rate is approximately 1 in 100,000 but geographical variations occur. The annual death rate for amyotrophic lateral sclerosis is 2.5/100,000, six times that of progressive muscular atrophy (0.4/100,000) but this difference may be partly due to the vagaries of certification and not reflect the true incidence of the two conditions (Norris & Kurland, 1969).

Age Incidence

Most patients present in the second half of life but the peak is in the fifth and seventh decades. Amyotrophic lateral sclerosis tends to occur at a slightly later age than progressive muscular atrophy (Table II).

TABLE II. Motor Neurone Disease (MND)

	PMA	ALS
Familial	–	+
Sex ratio	5 : 1	3 : 2
Age of onset	< 50 yrs	> 55 yrs
Fasciculation	–	++
Bulbar palsy	–	+
Average duration	> 6 yrs	< 4 yrs

MND = motor neurone disease; PMA = progressive muscular atrophy; ALS = amyotrophic lateral sclerosis

Sex Incidence

There is an overall majority in favour of the male in the proportion of 3 : 2. This is markedly exaggerated in progressive muscular atrophy (5 : 1) and reversed in bulbar palsy (2 : 3), although variations occur in different series (Table III).

TABLE III. Bulbar Palsy. Sex incidence

	♀	♂
Scheid, 1966	3	2
Sercl and Kovarik, 1967	3	2
Dozzi et al, 1969	3	2
Vejjajiva et al, 1972	1	1

2

Inheritance

Five to ten per cent of sporadic cases of MND are familial and they are thought to be transmitted as an autosomal dominant with variable penetrance. The sex ratio in these cases, as expected from this mode of transmission, is equal.

Geographical Inheritance

The cases found among the Chomorro tribe of Guam are identical with those occurring in the Kii peninsula of Japan, Filippinos in Hawaii and the Jaquai and Awjn tribes of Papua New Guinea. The disease occurs 100 times more frequently in Guam than elsewhere but differs in that the onset is earlier, especially in females, the course is slower even though the proportion presenting with bulbar symptoms is greater. It has been suggested that a neurotoxic cyanogenetic glycoside — cycadin — found in a Lathyrus-like fruit is responsible (see Chapter 2).

The pathology is different in that eosinophilic inclusions are commonly found, as are Alzheimer fibrillary changes. The latter are rare in sporadic MND but found in the brains of the Parkinsonian-Dementia syndrome, also seen in Guam. Twenty per cent of the latter develop MND and 10% of the Guamanian cases of MND develop the Parkinsonian-Dementia syndrome — a combination also seen outside the Mariana Islands.

Clinical Presentation and Prognosis

Most patients present with weakness of a limb but 30% will begin with bulbar palsy and more than 10% with a foot drop. The course is almost invariably progressive but more rapid in cases of bulbar palsy, where death occurs usually within three years. Most patients will on examination show both upper and lower motor neurone signs; cases of 'pure' progressive muscular atrophy in which there are no signs of an upper motor neurone lesion form less than 15% of most series and these patients often survive much longer than those with other variants.

When wasting begins in the hand, it affects first the thenar eminence; the thumb is then drawn back by the long extensor to produce a flat primate hand — 'main de singe'; later there is hyperextension of the metacarpophalangeal joints to produce a 'claw hand'. The disease will affect the forearm flexors, eg the biceps muscle, before the forearm extensors, eg the triceps muscle. Contrary to some opinion, the disease often has an asymmetrical onset and only later becomes symmetrical. The disease spreads up to the shoulders and can produce a 'wing-scapula'. The neck extensors may be early involved to produce a head drop — a proximal variety sometimes called the Vulpian-Bernhardt syndrome. When the head droops, the patient may need to hold it up with his hands; the cheeks become sunken but the frontalis muscles are not affected.

3

Fasciculation is, contrary to expectation, more often seen in ALS than in PMA. It may occur in any muscle but its diagnostic significance is increased if it is generalised or found in the tongue. The twitches may be felt by the patient and cramps can be a harbinger of the disease for months or even years before wasting is evident, often disappearing when wasting appears. Fasciculations can be increased by touch, percussion, compression or cold. They are usually limited to a motor unit but occasionally a synchronous discharge in many units takes place to produce a mass movement resembling a myoclonic jerk.

Upper motor neurone signs are usually present and this combination with atrophy and fasciculation is of great diagnostic significance. Although hyper-reflexia, hypertonia, and ankle clonus are not uncommon, a positive Babinski sign occurs in less than 20% of cases (Bonduelle, 1975). This is in contrast to other diseases where the upper motor neurone is involved, eg multiple sclerosis, when the positive Babinski is an early physical sign.

Unusual presentations include sensory symptoms and, very rarely, sensory signs. The external ocular muscles are rarely involved. Occasionally there is excessive fatiguability, suggestive of myasthenia; indeed, there may be a partial response to prostigmine — so-called 'pseudo-myasthenia'. This has been explained on the grounds that the regenerating motor-end plates produce defective neuro-muscular transmission.

BULBAR PALSY

There are two types, namely chronic bulbar palsy, where there is a LMN lesion and the condition is nearly always due to MND and pseudo-bulbar palsy where the UMN lesions are involved (Table IV). There are many causes of pseudo-

TABLE IV. Bulbar Palsy

	Chronic	Pseudo-
Dysarthria	+	+
Dysphagia	+	+
Tongue	Atrophy, fasciculation	Spasticity
Jaw jerk	−	++
Emotional lability	−	+

bulbar palsy, the commonest being cerebrovascular disease, but any bilateral UMN disease may produce the disease, eg multiple sclerosis, metastases.

Pseudobulbar palsy is less common than chronic bulbar palsy and, in addition to dysarthria, dysphonia and dysphagia (all of which are common to both) the glabellar and jaw jerks are brisk — indeed there may be clonus of

TABLE V. Motor Neurone Disease. Bulbar Presentation

	N	Bulbar presentation
Mustova, 1971	77	29%
Nishigaki, 1972	133	37%
Muller-Jensen & Bernhardt, 1973	226	25%

the jaw — and there is emotional lability. This takes the form of pathological laughter or crying, not necessarily associated with change of mood. Pathological laughter can be prolonged; it is often provoked by rapid drinking and can be arrested by deep breathing. The tongue is spastic, ie it moves slowly and as a whole mass rather than independent movements within the tongue. About one-third of patients with MND present with bulbar palsy (Table V).

Speech

Since it is estimated that more than 100 muscles are involved in speaking, it is not surprising that a disturbance of speech is the earliest sign but this is more likely to be noticed by others than the patient. As the earliest facial muscle to be involved is the orbicularis oris, it is the bilabial plosives — 'p' and 'b' — that are first affected. For the same reason, the patient has early difficulty in whistling. With weakness of the soft palate there is a nasal sound to speech — hyperrhinolalia — due to nasal escape of air. The soft palate may hang down and be immobile so that there is regurgitation of fluids through the nose; the palatal weakness is usually, but not invariably, symmetrical. The lower jaw droops and there is salivation, particularly in the pseudo-bulbar variety. Patients may complain that the tongue is heavy or tired and examination will reveal that it is flaccid, atrophic and fibrillating. Dysphonia is often present and may be due to weakness of the respiratory musculature; this tends to occur later in the disease when the intercostal muscles may be sunken and the diaphragm paralysed.

Because of a superior laryngeal palsy, the vocal cords are no longer tense and this produces a hoarseness and, because of lack of modulation, the voice is monotonous.

With bilateral recurrent laryngeal palsy, the vocal cords are in a paramedian position and Semon's law is not rigidly followed. An early presentation of dysphonia due to laryngeal paralysis may be surprisingly acute in onset. Immobile cords produce a rough, rasping or 'fricative' quality to the speech. The patient may complain of dyspnoea, and choking will occur because rigidity of the glottis prevents closure of the larynx during swallowing.

Patients will speak slowly and choose their words carefully to avoid too obvious dysarthria and speech is even slower in the pseudo-bulbar variety.

The monotonous voice is not specific (since it occurs commonly in Parkin-

5

sonism) but it is more frequently heard in the pseudo-bulbar variety. Speech tends to fade in intensity at the end of the sentence. In the majority of cases, the singing voice is eventually lost. In a later stage, the patient may not be able to clear the mouth and larynx and retained mucus produces a gurgling or bubbly sound to speech. A compensation mechanism for tongue paralysis is to raise the jaw.

In the pseudobulbar variety, speech is not only slow, but sentences are short. Consonants are indistinct, there are alterations in pitch and phonation, and intensity (loudness) is reduced. Nasal speech occurs both in this variety and progressive bulbar palsy where the dysarthria is mixed, ie there is both progressive bulbar and pseudobulbar palsy present; not only are the intervals between sentences and words longer, but the phonemes themselves are prolonged; there is altered phrasing with grunts at the end of sentences (Colmant, 1975).

Swallowing

Progressive bulbar palsy may present with dysphagia, often aggravated by alcohol. Normally, the orbicularis oris muscle holds the food bolus before the floor of the mouth is lowered and the tongue presses the bolus against the hard palate to reduce its size; it is then pushed back to the posterior pharyngeal wall to initiate the swallowing reflex. All these muscles may be affected in progressive bulbar palsy, although some movements may be more affected than others. Paralysis of the muscles of mastication may affect biting and grinding movements differentially but eventually the jaw droops and there is difficulty in swallowing saliva. The tongue may fall backwards necessitating a change in head positions; when completely paralysed the bolus of food may have to be pushed back manually.

During the pharyngo-oesophageal phase of the swallowing reflex (under the control of a medullary centre) the glottis closes and breathing reflex ceases; the upper third of the oesophagus has striated muscle in its wall but the further swallowing in the lower two-thirds is served by an intramural reflex (at the rate of 4 cm/sec). This may be abnormal in MND and produce a reflux oesophagitis. In addition to decreased oesophageal mobility, there may be dilatation of the stomach as well as cardiac, respiratory and vestibular involvement.

The nasopharynx is closed off by the action of the palatal levator and tensor muscles as well as the constrictor muscles of the superior larynx. If the latter are paralysed, when the patient takes a breath following swallowing, the bolus, retained in the pharynx because of pharyngeal stasis, enters the larynx. This is the commonest mode of death in progressive bulbar palsy. Besides asphyxia, other causes of death include aspiration pneumonia, inanition and cardiac failure. Death usually occurs within two-and-a-half years of onset of progressive bulbar, irrespective of age of onset. There are several associations with bulbar palsy (see Table VI).

TABLE VI. Bulbar Palsy Associations

1	Familial spastic paraplegia
2	Huntington's chorea
3	Dementia (Pick's, parkinsonism – dementia complex)
4	Progressive supranuclear palsy (Steele-Richardson-Olszewski syndrome)
5	Autonomic nervous disease
	(a) Shy-Drager syndrome
	(b) Riley-Day syndrome
6	Deafness in children (vestibular and cerebellar signs and optic atrophy)
7	Corneal dystrophy
8	External ophthalmoplegia
9	Palatal myoclonus
10	Neoplasms

Effort dyspnoea may be an early sign of MND. Respiratory involvement may be due to paralysis of the intercostal muscles and diaphragm which may produce paradoxical movements. The vital capacity is reduced, there is hypoventilation with reduced pO_2 (Colmant, 1975).

DIFFERENTIAL DIAGNOSIS

Wasting of the Hand

This may be due to a spinal cord lesion involving the anterior horn cells as in syringomyelia but the characteristic dissociated anaesthesia will be found. Peripheral nerve lesions can be recognised by the distribution of the wasting, eg a

TABLE VII. Hand Wasting

1	Peripheral nerve lesion (ulnar)
2	Peripheral neuropathy (feet involved)
3	PMA (often asymmetrical onset)
4	Trauma (plexus or root – C8 T1)
5	Cervical rib (rare)
6	Syringomyelia (dissociated anaesthesia)

median nerve lesion will affect the thenar eminence whereas the latter will be spared in an ulnar nerve lesion; the appropriate sensory loss can also be determined. An X-ray of the neck may need to be done to exclude a cervical rib or, more rarely a cause of hand wasting, spondylosis (Table VII).

Spastic Paraplegia

The two commonest causes for this would be cervical cord compression, as in spondylosis, or multiple sclerosis. The latter usually affects a younger age group and should present little difficulty if there is the dissemination of space and time. Cervical spondylosis, however, may be very difficult to distinguish and, indeed, the two conditions not uncommonly occur together.

Bulbar Palsy

Possibly the next commonest cause of this would be bilateral strokes or cerebral arteriosclerosis but there would be no evidence of a lower motor neurone lesion such as wasting or fasciculation of the tongue in this case. Myasthenia would be

TABLE VIII. Aetiology of Bulbar Palsy

1	Bilateral strokes
2	MND
3	MS
4	Bilateral tumours
5	Syringobulbia
6	Myasthenia
7	Myopathy

characterised by increasing dysarthria when the patient speaks or dysphagia as he chews and a Tensilon test will confirm the diagnosis. Myopathy may also need to be considered (Table VIII).

Foot Drop

Possibly the commonest cause of this would be a lateral popliteal palsy or pro-lapsed disc but in the latter there may be some history of back pain and in both there is usually sensory loss which is not found in motor neurone disease. Poly-neuritis would present with bilateral foot drop and again there would be the characteristic distal sensory loss as well as areflexia. A lesion of the conus or cauda equina must also be considered (Table IX).

TABLE IX. Foot Drop

1	Lateral popliteal palsy
2	Prolapsed intervertebral disc
3	MND
4	Polyneuritis
5	Conus or cauda equina lesion

Proximal limb weakness can be due to polymositis but the EMG and biopsy will usually solve any clinical doubts.

Fasciculation may be seen in thyrotoxic myopathy but the appropriate endocrine investigations with I^{131} will determine its presence. Benign fasciculation is not rare, especially in young medical students, but there will be no evidence of denervation electrophysiologically.

INVESTIGATIONS

The clinical diagnosis, particularly in the more advanced case, is usually all too obvious but because of the poor prognosis it is important to exclude other conditions.

(a)   Perhaps the most important investigation is electromyography. Spontaneous denervation activity with fibrillation potentials and positive sharp waves are often seen. The fasciculations seen clinically are represented electrically by motor unit discharges. The maximum voluntary action pattern is reduced and there may be high amplitude potentials (see Chapter 11).

(b)   Lumbar puncture is most helpful in excluding other conditions. In motor neurone disease there is occasionally a slight rise in CSF protein, particularly in PMA and the gamma globulin is raised in 30% of cases.

(c)   Muscle biopsy will confirm the presence of denervation and re-innervation by showing group atrophy of muscle fibres (see Chapter 8).

TREATMENT

It is important that food should be chewed slowly and be given in semi-solid or pureed form. Food should be given at the lowest temperature and carefully chewed so that meals will be necessarily prolonged. Head positioning is important, especially during sleep.

Prostigmine and strychnine will help swallowing and there is no doubt that tracheostomy, sometimes with assisted ventilation, and gastrostomy will prolong life (or the act of dying?). Salivation can be helped by anti-cholinergic drugs and has also been treated by radiotherapy to, or removal of, the salivary glands, ligation of salivary ducts or cutting the chorda tympani and tympanic nerves. The latter moreover reduces saliva by 95% and does not cause xerostomia but will produce ageusia.

With the speechless patient, several ingenious attempts at communication methods have been tried, eg a small lamp on the forehead directed to an alphabetic board at the end of the bed; use of Morse Code pips, which can be converted into a text, or even an electropharynx. It should be remembered that intellect is preserved and these patients should be spoken to normally.

There are diseases related to those already described in this chapter which do not have the same clinical pattern. Because the pathological basis lies in the motor neurone, they have been included under the rubric of 'motor neurone diseases'

TABLE X. Motor Neurone Diseases

1	MND	a) ALS
		b) PMA
		c) Bulbar palsy
2	Werdnig-Hoffman (Infantile MA)	
3	Kugelberg-Welander (Proximal MA)	
4	Juvenile bulbar palsy	
5	Others	

(Table X). It should be emphasised that the prognosis varies considerably from group to group.

Werdnig-Hoffman Syndrome

The name given to infantile spinal muscular atrophy, it is inherited as in an auto-somal recessive manner but it is suggested that two genes are involved, ie there is an 'activator' gene.

It has been suggested there are two main types: an acute form manifesting before the age of six months and resulting in death within three years and a more chronic form where the disease appears to start after the age of one year and survival continues into the second decade but with marked disablement. Sucking and swallowing is poor, the face lacks expression, the jaw hangs down and the tongue is atrophied and fasciculating and speech is nasal; there is also atrophy of the facial and sternomastoid muscles. There is involvement of the

TABLE XI. The Floppy Infant

1	Benign hypotonia	
2	Cerebral palsy	
3	Congenital myopathies	a) muscular dystrophy
		b) Pompe's disease
		c) Others
4	Dystrophia myotonica	
5	Myasthenia	
6	Metachromatic leucodystrophy	
7	Werdnig-Hoffman	
8	Systemic –	Down's syndrome
		endocrine,
		trauma

10

trunk as well as cervical musculature and the baby adopts the 'frog' position, with limbs abducted and not moving. Fasciculation is rarely seen in the limbs, possibly because of the presence of subcutaneous fat. There is generalised tendon areflexia. The initial presentation in the majority of cases is either as arthyrogryposis congenita or a 'floppy baby' (Table XI).

In Werdnig-Hoffman syndrome, the muscle enzymes are usually normal and the myopathic changes in biopsy specimens are less than in the Kugelberg-Welander Syndrome. The EMG in this condition shows a unique feature in relaxed muscles of a 5–15 c/sec motor unit activity, discharging regularly. Nearly all patients with Kugelberg-Welander will survive into the second decade, and still be able to walk (Table XII).

TABLE XII.

	Werdnig-Hoffman	Kugelberg-Welander
Inheritance	Autosomal recessive	Any type
Age of presentation	<1 yr	>1 yr
Mode of presentation	'Floppy infant'	'Muscular dystrophy'
Wasting	Face, neck, trunk	Proximal limbs
Fasciculation	Tongue	Limbs (50%)
Unable to walk	<10 yrs	>10 yrs
Survival	3–10 yrs	20 yrs

Kugelberg-Welander Syndrome

Although MND usually begins in the distal limb musculature and runs a progressive course, there is a group of patients – and nearly 400 have been reported in the literature – where disease affects the proximal limb musculature and runs a much slower course. In this regard it clinically resembles muscular dystrophy but just over twenty years ago, with the help of electromyography, it was shown to be neurogenic in origin (Kugelberg & Welander, 1954; Wohlfart et al, 1958).

Also called juvenile pseudo-myopathic spinal muscular atrophy, this syndrome is not always distinguishable from the Werdnig-Hoffman syndrome. Nearly 30% have bulbar involvement and there may be ptosis, facial and sternomastoid weakness with tongue fasciculation.

Age of Onset

Although the condition may be seen at any age, there are two peak ages of presentation as nearly half the cases occur between the ages of 3 and 18 (juvenile) and over one-third before the age of 2 years (infantile). The age of onset seems

11

to be similar within families. Its commonest mode of inheritance is autosomal recessive but it can be dominant with incomplete or irregular penetrance or sex-linked.

Sex Incidence

There is a predominance of males, particularly in those with a later onset.

Presenting Symptoms

This usually starts with delay or difficulty in walking but the upper limb girdle becomes affected years later, and its neurogenic origin can be recognised clinically by the presence of fasciculation in about half the cases, and better seen in males than females because of less subcutaneous fat. The weakness and wasting is proximal and symmetrical, as with muscular dystrophy, and the same features of winged scapula, lordosis, waddling gait and Gower's sign (climbing up the thighs from the prone position) are present. The patient cannot lift his head from the pillow but can sit up.

Investigations

Raised muscle enzyme levels are present in half the cases, but not to the same degree as found in muscular dystrophy. Electromyography shows the characteristics of chronic denervation, viz reduced interference pattern and large motor unit potentials due to collateral reinnervation producing increased fibre density; insertion activity, spontaneous fibrillation potentials and positive sharp spikes are much less common than in MND. Muscle biopsy also shows the characteristic changes of denervation with small angular fibres and loss of checker-board appearance, type grouping and group atrophy. Myopathic changes of variation in fibre size, fibre splitting, central nucleation and interstitial tissue increases can also be seen.

References

Aran, FA (1850) *Archives of General Medicine, 24,* 15, 172
Bell, C (1830) *The Nervous System of the Human Body.* Longman, London
    Pages 132 and 160
Bonduelle, M (1975) *Handbook of Clinical Neurology, Vol.22.* (Ed) PJ Vinken
    and GW Bruyn. North Holland Publishing Co, London. Page 281
Charcot, J-M (1873) *Lecons sur les maladies du systeme nerveux, II me series.*
    Delaheuxe, Paris. Page 192
Colmant, HJ (1975) *Handbook of Clinical Neurology, Vol.22.* (Ed) PJ Vinken
    and GW Bruyn. North Holland Publishing Co, London. Page 111
Dazzi, P, Finizio, FS and Mercuriali, A (1969) *Giornale di psichiatria e di
    neuropatologia, 97,* 711

Duchenne, G (1860) *Archives of General Medicine, 16,* 283, 431

Kugelberg, E and Welander, C (1954) *Acta psychiatrica et neurologica Scandinavica, 29,* 42

Muller-Jensen, A and Bernhardt, W (1973) *Nervenarzt, 44,* 143

Musatova, IV (1971) *Zhurnal nevropatologil i psykhiatril i neni SS Korsakova, 71,* 574

Nighigaki, S (1972) *Arzneimittel-Forschung, 26,* 402

Norris, FH and Kurland, LT (1969) *Motor Neuron Diseases.* Grune and Stratton, London

Scheid, W (1966) *Lehrbuch der Neurologie, 2nd impr.* Georg Thieme, Stuttgart. Page 508

Sercl, M and Kovarik, J (1967) *Sbornik vedeckych praci Lekarske fakulty Karlovy university v Hradci Kralove, 10,* 411

Vejjajiva, A, Forster, JB and Miller, H (1972) *Journal of Neurological Sciences, 4,* 299

Wohlfart, A, Fex, J and Eliasson, S (1955) *Acta psychiatrica et neurologica Scandinavica, 30,* 395

CHAPTER TWO

EPIDEMIOLOGY OF AMYOTROPHIC LATERAL SCLEROSIS, WITH EMPHASIS ON ANTECEDENT EVENTS FROM CASE-CONTROL COMPARISONS

Leonard T Kurland

In the past few years, the descriptive epidemiology of motor neurone disease (MND) has received several comprehensive reviews (Kurland et al, 1969; Bobo-wick & Brody, 1973; Brody & Kurland, 1973; Kurland et al, 1973). These are largely in agreement with respect to the incidence, geographical distribution, and population characteristics of amyotrophic lateral sclerosis (ALS) and other components of motor neurone disease. However, there have been relatively few analytical studies aimed at clarifying aetiology; and almost all of these have been limited to observational data on possible risk factors in series of patients — only a few comparative studies of cases and controls have been reported.

It is my intent to present a working definition of epidemiology and to define ALS as a component of motor neurone disease; then (1) to review, briefly, the highlights of the geographical distribution and population selectivity of ALS; (2) to describe methods and problems of data collection and data analysis in case-control studies; and, (3) to discuss aetiological possibilities rendered plausible by the results of clinical, family, and community studies.

Working Definition of Epidemiology

Epidemiology is concerned with the frequency, geographical distribution, and population dynamics of disease which may be helpful in aetiology and disease control.

Methodologically, after the clinical, pathological and familial description of cases and case series are presented, population-based studies may develop. Analyses of mortality data provide a broad picture of disease distribution; morbidity surveys may then be designed to identify those subpopulations prone to, and free from, the disease by age, sex, race, etc. Retrospective case control comparisons may then be designed to search for possible causative factors. If case control studies are successful in identifying one or more factors that appear to be aetiologically associated with the disease, a prospective study of the suspected factor may be tried if ethical requirements for such an experiment can be fulfilled.

Since there are indications that, for ALS, some host factors (endogenous mechanisms) and those of the environment may be interrelated aetiologically, the epidemiologist should also be able to determine familial aggregation and provide basic genetic analyses of such data.

Definition of ALS

The term 'motor neurone disease' refers to progressive involvement of upper or lower motor neurones, usually with little or no clinical involvement of sensory or other non-motor tracts. ALS is a major component of MND; and as used by many neurologists in the United States, 'ALS' is a term of convenience that includes progressive muscular atrophy (with its primary abnormality in the anterior horn cells) and progressive bulbar palsy (with analogous changes in the motor cranial-nerve nuclei). To fit this definition, the lower motor neurones must be affected: upper motor neurone lesions manifested by 'lateral sclerosis' and 'pseudo-bulbar palsy' need not be present. In most cases that are diagnosed initially as progressive muscular atrophy or progressive bulbar palsy and come to autopsy, upper motor neurone lesions are found.

As used here, ALS will comprise a group of disorders with onset in adult life and with predominant clinical and pathological evidence of disease of the motor neurones. Weakness and atrophy of muscles are apparent, often with fasciculations and EMG evidence of denervation. Conduction velocities are usually normal and sensation and mentation are seldom affected. The rate of involvement of the pyramidal tract determines the extent to which muscle stretch reflexes are diminished or enhanced and whether pathological reflexes are observed.

In the International Classification of Diseases, primary lateral sclerosis unfortunately is included under the motor neurone disease rubric. In my opinion, primary lateral sclerosis should be in a distinct category. However, in most countries this syndrome accounts for only a very small fraction of the deaths under the motor neurone disease rubric and does not seriously affect comparisons of mortality rates.

DESCRIPTIVE EPIDEMIOLOGY OF ALS

Patterns of Incidence

This includes the study of the geographical distribution by age, sex, race, etc. ALS has been recognised in every country in which there is neurological expertise. Because mortality data for ALS in the developed countries are reasonably accurate and are readily available, they serve as a substitute for incidence rates, since the disease seems to be invariably fatal and no appreciable difference in duration of life after onset has been noted by region or by major types of the disease.

Study of the geographical pattern based on mortality rates reveals that such rates are remarkably similar in the developed countries of Western Europe and North America and in Australia, New Zealand, and Japan. Among these nations it accounts for about 1/1,000 adult deaths and the age-adjusted rate approaches 1/100,000 population per year (Kurland et al, 1969).

In the United States, death rates for ALS and progressive muscular atrophy (PMA) combined have increased only slightly in the past 25 years; within this grouping, the proportion of deaths assigned to ALS has increased steadily from 60% to more than 80% of the total, as PMA-designated deaths have decreased correspondingly, This shift probably reflects increasing physician preference for the former term. rather than any change in the MND characteristics in the nation.

In the United States there is no appreciable selectivity by state or region (Kurland et al, 1973), degree of urbanisation, marital status, or nativity (native vs foreign born). Although the reported rate is higher in whites than in non-whites (1.7 : 1), it is uncertain whether this reflects a true difference in incidence or is related to the availability and utilisation of diagnostic services. In Rochester, Minnesota, where the records-linkage system of the Mayo Clinic provides unusually complete data on the local population, there has been a slight, not statistically significant, upward trend in the incidence over the past three decades. The mean annual incidence rate in Rochester has been about 1.6/100,000 (age-adjusted to the US 1950 population). The incidence rates for recent years in Iceland and in Carlisle, England are about 1/100,000 per year (Kurland et al, 1973).

On the basis of the Rochester (Minnesota) and national mortality data, it is estimated that in the United States about 3,000 to 4,000 new cases occur annually and about 12,000 to 16,000 persons are affected with ALS at any given time. The corresponding incidence and prevalence in the United Kingdom would be about 1,000 and 4,000 cases.

The mean age at onset in the small series of cases in Rochester, Minnesota was about 64 years, which contrasts with about 53 years in several clinical series. The national mortality data for the United States indicate that the mean age at death for both males and females is about 62 years (Kurland et al, 1969). Since the mean duration from onset to death is about 4 years, this suggests that the mean age at onset derived from clinical series (53 years) may be incorrect, since clinical series – particularly those from specialty services or hospitals – often have an inherent bias toward selection of younger patients. It is suggested that the mean age at onset for ALS may be closer to 60 years.

The remarkable foci of ALS among the Chamorro population of the Mariana Islands and among Japanese in a rather isolated area on Honshu known as the Kii Peninsula stand out in contrast to the remarkably similar rates reported from the rest of Japan and other well developed countries (Kurland & Mulder, 1954;

16

Kimura et al, 1963; Yase et al, 1968). In most villages within these foci the incidence rate for ALS is about 50 to 100 times that reported in other parts of the world.

Particularly in the Marianas, there is also prevalent an unusual form of neurological illness characterised by progressive dementia, basal ganglia disease, and upper motor neurone involvement which is referred to as the Parkinsonism-Dementia Complex (PD) (Hirano et al, 1961). About 20% of the patients with PD subsequently develop the lower motor neurone disease of ALS as well. It was the recognition of the neurofibrillary changes and granulovacuolar bodies (intracytoplasmic inclusions) in the neurones of the PD patients that led to identification of the same distinctive histological features in the ALS of the Mariana Islands and some of the cases in the Kii Peninsula (Hirano et al, 1961; Shiraki & Yase, 1975). The age and sex distributions, the frequent occurrence of both disorders in the same patient, the familial pattern of ALS and PD, and the similarity of histological findings in affected neurones support the view that PD in the Marianas (and possibly Kii) is a clinical variant of the ALS which occurs in this region. Similar histological changes, although of a lesser degree, have also been found in about half of the adult Chamorros over age 45 who do not have obvious ALS or PD at time of death (Anderson et al, 1976). This suggests that the common basis of these diseases and perhaps of a subclinical variant of *forme fruste* of the Western Pacific type of ALS may be the neurofibrillary changes.

Although ALS and PD originally were noted only in the Chamorros of Guam and the other Mariana Islands, several cases have occurred in recent years among Filipinos on Guam and among other groups. However, most of these did not have the pathological hallmark noted among the Chamorros (Stanhope et al, 1972).

Filipinos in Hawaii appear to have an increased incidence of ALS, but apparently do not show the neurofibrillary changes. Little or no information is available about the prevalence or characteristics of ALS in the areas of the Philippine Islands from which they came (Matsumoto et al, 1972).

ALS was not noted to any increased extent in the population of the Caroline Islands in the nearby Trust Territories (Kurland & Mulder, 1955). A search for ALS among the small number of adult descendents of the Chamorros from Saipan who were transferred to New Britain early in this century also failed to disclose any cases of ALS in that group. ALS is prevalent among Guamanian immigrants to the continental United States, but it is still too early to determine whether the rate will diminish in the generation born on the mainland.

Since 1965, it appears, the incidence rates for ALS and PD have been declining appreciably on Guam (Reed & Brody, 1975). Because genetic factors cannot readily explain that change, an exogenous basis for this focus of ALS seems most likely (as remarked in the section on Aetiological Considerations in this chapter).

17

Forms of ALS

Three forms of ALS can be identified on the basis of their clinical, pathological, and epidemiological characteristics. These are referred to as (1) sporadic or classical, (2) familial and presumably hereditary, and (3) the Mariana Island form — perhaps more appropriately the Western Pacific Islands type.

Classical or Sporadic Form

About 90 to 95% of the cases observed in the United States occur as a singular event in a family and have the classical features of progressive lower motor neurone disease, usually with evidence of upper neurone involvement. Most patients are in the fifth to seventh decades; although clinical series suggest the mean age at onset is about 53 years, for reasons stated above it probably approximates 60 years. The preponderance in males, about 1.6 : 1, is unexplained.

The site of initial wasting and weakness varies; but in most series is described as the upper extremity in about 40%, bulbar level and lower extremity in about 25% each, and mixed in about 10%. Pathologically, there is neuronal loss in the anterior horns and demyelination of the anterolateral tracts, especially the pyramidal tracts; these changes usually contrast sharply with the well-preserved surrounding tissues. In the brain stem also, motor nuclei and pyramids may be affected but are usually surrounded by intact structures (Hirano et al, 1969).

Dermal changes that include increased mucopolysaccharides, connective-tissue disorientation, elastosis, and disorganisation of collagen structure are believed to reflect a possible biochemical defect. These were noted in about 50% of a group of sporadic cases studied in the United States and significantly less often in a control group (Fullmer et al, 1960).

Familial Form

On the basis of several series reported from the Mayo Clinic and elsewhere it appears that about 5 to 10% of ALS cases occur in a familial pattern that is compatible with a dominant trait. Although the individual case of this kind has no distinctive feature detectable on clinical examination, it appears that a relatively high proportion of such cases begin with weakness and wasting in the lower extremities and that progression is fairly rapid. Hirano and associates (1969) described the neuropathological features observed, including clinically silent involvement of the mid-root zone of the posterior columns and involvement of the spinocerebellar tracts and loss of cells in Clarke's column, and presence of hyalin-like material within the cytoplasma of affected anterior horn cells.

Such cases may represent a transitional type in the genetic spectrum that encompasses the hereditary ataxias and ALS. Other familial cases, particularly those with initial cervical or bulbar involvement, have shown nothing distinctive pathologically and appear to be identical to the classic or sporadic cases.

The familial cases show a 1 : 1 sex ratio, contrasting with the male preponderance observed in the classical and Mariana Islands form. Histochemical changes in the skin have not been seen in the few familial cases that have been studied.

Although the mean age at onset is perhaps 10 years less than in the sporadic cases, the range of onset ages is wide (Kurland & Mulder, 1955). Members of some families develop the disease at about the same age, whereas in other families it may vary by 20 or 30 years. A very late age of onset may account for the apparent occasional 'skipped generation'. In 1959 Engel, Klatzo and I described a family in which the mother of two patients with ALS (onset in the fourth and fifth decades) was living and well at age 68. This lady's brother had died of ALS at age 57, so it appeared that she had transmitted the gene without being affected herself. Not until the age of 81 years did she develop symptoms of progressive weakness. At autopsy "the changes of amyotrophic lateral sclerosis were apparent microscopically and were seen in the region of the hypoglossal nucleus, the Betz cells . . . . Also present was . . . . a bronchiolar (alveolar cell) type neoplasm and . . . . a non-encapsulating sclerosing carcinoma of the thyroid . . . . in none of these lesions was extension or metastasis demonstrated." (Alpert et al, 1972).

The relationship of bronchogenic carcinoma to amyotrophy is still uncertain (Norris et al, 1969), and whether it has some special significance in the familial form remains to be seen.

Marianas (Western Pacific) Form

In the individual case, the Marianas form cannot be distinguished clinically from the sporadic form (Kurland & Mulder, 1955). Although the range of onset age is similar to that of the sporadic cases, the mean is several years less. Males predominate by about 2 : 1. The mean duration of the disease (approximately 4 years) and the major pathological features (anterior horn cell degeneration and demyelination of the long motor tracts) do not differ from those of the sporadic form. However, neurofibrillary changes and granulovacuolar bodies, which are observed infrequently elsewhere, are common in the Marianas form of the disease. I consider PD a clinical variant of the Marianas type of ALS. The neurofibrillary changes which are so common among the Chamorros may reflect widespread exposure to some still unidentified toxic agent. The histochemical changes in the skin noted in the sporadic cases were also noted in about half the Guam ALS and PD cases studied (Fullmer et al, 1960).

RETROSPECTIVE CASE CONTROL COMPARISONS

Several different studies of ALS have provided an accumulation of clinical, pathological, and genetic data, international mortality statistics, mortality rates for each state in the United States, and incidence rates and familial patterns in

Rochester (Minnesota), the Marianas, and the Kii Peninsula. These proceeded methodically but slowly over a difficult 10-year period of research that is described in the history of the Epidemiology Branch, NINDB (Kurland & Brody, 1975).

The assembled information led to the designation of at least three apparently distinct forms of ALS. Since the prevalence of ALS is low and the possible aetiological factors are many, retrospective or case control studies seem to be warranted.

Some of the earlier studies of ALS cases (which will be reviewed) included laboratory tests for heavy metals and other agents and inquiries about possible risk factors; but in many the results are not suitable for comparison. Since there are numerous possibilities of bias in such unilateral investigations, some of the reports have been received with scepticism, although they might serve as a guide for subsequent studies of cases and controls.

In the early stages of the research programme on Guam in the late 1950s, familial studies and some case control comparisons were initiated; but the latter were not particularly enlightening (Reed et al, 1966; Plato et al, 1969). The well designed studies by Reed et al (1955, 1975) recently reported have produced considerable data that should help narrow the search for the presumed aetiological agents or mechanism of the Marianas form of ALS. But before taking up a summary of their results and those of other recent case control studies, it seems appropriate to consider the methods of such retrospective efforts and the problems inherent in them. The primary source of the comments that follow is the excellent section on medical surveys in *Statistics in Medicine* by Colton (1974), which also covers cross-sectional and prospective study methods that will not be discussed here.

In a retrospective study, the investigator identifies a group of patients and — as a standard of comparison — a 'control' group without the disease. For each case and control, the investigator obtains a history of the presence or absence of a risk factor or the degree of exposure to such a factor. If there is sufficient evidence that the risk factor is present more frequently or occurs at a higher level among cases than controls, the investigator may conclude that there is an association between the risk factor and the disease.

The case control method is feasible for studying diseases of low incidence, because cases can be collected in a large referral centre or through multi-centre collaboration. Many different risk factors can be included in the inquiry, and it is possible to perform such screening studies rapidly and at fairly low cost.

The disadvantages of the case control method include uncertainty of the representativeness of the sample (or selection) of the patients and the accuracy and completeness of retrospective inquiry on risk factors that may be remote in time. Also the presence of the disease may influence recollection of the factor being studied.

As Colton remarked, "Three critical aspects of retrospective studies deserve attention: (a) the criteria employed for definition of cases and identification of the factor under study, (2) the selection of controls and their comparability with the cases, and (3) the accuracy of the histories of exposure to the risk factors."

1. Obviously, every effort should be made to ensure that the cases accepted as instances of the disease are indeed that. Cases of ALS should fulfil criteria such as those given at the beginning of this paper; and a decision must be made to include the uncommon form with only lower motor neurone disease or to restrict the series to cases with both upper and lower motor neurone involvement. Furthermore, it seems most important to deal separately with the three forms of ALS referred to earlier, since it is likely that the aetiology of each may be distinct, even though in time the basic pathological mechanism may prove to be similar in all three types.

It is also important that the cases included in the study be a fair representation of all cases, unselected in regard to exposure to the risk factors under study.

2. In the selection of controls, the goal is to obtain controls as similar as possible to the patients with respect to such variables as age, sex, and race — the obvious difference being only the presence or absence of the disease in question. Two methods are available: matched pairs and stratified random sampling from the community. Each has its advantages.

The matching variables which might be considered involve the use of siblings, spouses, those who shared the childhood environment or those who share the adult or an occupational environment. A good way to avoid overmatching is to match on little else except current neighbourhood environment. Neighbourhood controls of the same age, race, and sex have some distinct methodological advantages and are generally easy to obtain. A general principle is that variables one wishes to evaluate should not be used in the matching. In developing suitable matches for ALS,,the list of variables under study is so broad that one or another would exclude several of the methods of matches suggested above. In items dealing with childhood environment, the use of sibling controls would be an inefficient method since siblings ordinarily would not differ on these items. It appears that, after identification of the type of ALS to be studied, only age, sex, and race may be appropriate variables for matching and that the neighbourhood control may prove to be the most useful.

Since factors from the childhood environment may be causes of the disease, it seems that, for some ALS studies at least, stratified random sampling from the community would be preferable to matching, although perhaps more difficult. Such a control procedure was used in the recently reported studies on Guam (Reed et al, 1966; Reed & Brody, 1975).

3. In retrospective studies it is important that the data concerning presence of risk factors be sought in the same manner among cases and controls, whether by interview or by review of records. If a prevailing clinical impression has already led to a more intensive inquiry and recording of the risk factor in the patients than in the controls, the possibility of spurious association of a risk factor must be kept in mind.

21

Although case control comparison may establish an association between the risk factor and the disease, the magnitude of the difference in risk cannot be estimated directly. However, in most studies the conditions are such that it is possible to get an indirect estimate of the ratio of the two risks in the cases and in the controls, ie the relative risk.

When the comparison is made between individuals in matched pairs, those pairs wherein exposure of the case and control is equal contribute no information. The effective sample size then is the number of untied pairs. When the comparison is between two groups selected independently (eg randomised, stratified population samples vs cases), the sample size is the total number of persons studied. However, the question of which method is more powerful in detecting association between disease and risk factors cannot be answered in general, since the exposure rates and the efficiency of the matching must be taken into consideration.

AETIOLOGICAL CONSIDERATIONS

There is evidence of at least three major forms of ALS (sporadic or classical, Marianas, familial and presumably hereditary forms). There may even be more than one familial and presumably hereditary type. The underlying and precipitating causes of these types are conceivably quite different, and studies and analyses performed should take the different types into consideration.

In the study of aspects such as the immune state, it is difficult at this juncture to decide whether a feature such as the increased proportion of patients with a specific HLA type reflects presence of a simple genetic variant, or whether deposition of some immune complex implies an increased likelihood of a CNS disease in response to some infectious or toxic agent. Nevertheless, certain of these features are more conveniently, albeit arbitrarily, discussed under the heading of 'familial form' and others under 'sporadic form'.

Familial Form

The familial form in adults, as described earlier (Kurland & Mulder, 1955), appears to be transmitted as a dominant trait. Common exposure of generation after generation of the same family to the same infectious, traumatic, or toxic precipitating episodes in a pattern resembling that of dominant inheritance appears highly unlikely; so search for an underlying metabolic abnormality seems to be a more reasonable approach.

Since ALS is an infrequent occurrence and the familial form accounts for less than 10% of cases, the collection of a sizeable series of living patients with the presumably hereditary disease may require collaboration among referral centres. Large numbers are required by the assumption that the difference between cases and controls may not be clearcut: quantitative data from the two groups may overlap, or the answers to a crucial question about antecedent events may not be obviously different.

Among the metabolic mechanisms to be considered is a histochemical change in the collagen of skin and the mucopolysaccharide content. Negative findings in familial cases have been reported by Fullmer et al (1960), but the observations were very few. An appropriate search might include repetition of such studies in affected families and efforts to refine the techniques, since the skin is one of the few tissues readily available for direct examination during life.

Although one might speculate from experience with pernicious anaemia that the underlying metabolic defect occurs outside the nervous system, there is, as yet, no adequate basis for that assumption. Mulder and I have seen one family with stomach cancer or ALS in several members and more than one generation, but repeated and systematic studies would be more convincing than such clinical observations.

Reports of an ALS-like condition following gastrectomy or in conjunction with hypoglycaemia and possibly pancreatic abnormalities have been reviewed by Norris (1976), but he concluded that the low incidence of measurable changes in his own large series of ALS suggests an incidental rather than an aetiological relationship. However, such analyses are yet to be reported in a sizeable series of familial cases.

Since autolysis — which may blur seemingly minor changes in the liver, pancreas, and other organs — occurs so rapidly after death, needle biopsy or prompt postmortem examination should be considered as means of obtaining tissue for appropriate morphological, histochemical, and electron microscopic studies to detect change, if it is indeed present in such tissues outside the central nervous system.

Immunological studies may detect inherent differences as well as enhanced responses to some exogenous agent. There may be value in further studies such as those by Oldstone et al (1973), where immunofluorescence in renal glomerular biopsies revealed IgG and the third component of complement (C3). Norris (1974) notes that the deposits did not stain for poliovirus types $1-3$, human myelin, or myelin basic protein; so there is no substantial clue as to whether they indicate a host-virus encounter or an epiphenomenon such as the circulation of by-products from cell degeneration.

No consistent pattern has been discovered in attempts to identify a distinct HLA type in ALS. Arnason (1976) has noted a higher prevalence in cases than in controls for locus A-3 and possibly B-12, but the number of cases is small and the variety of types is large. More studies must be completed, and some discrimination by type of ALS may also be appropriate.

Marianas (Western Pacific) Form

In recent years the patterns of ALS and PD have been restudied for patterns of

23

geography over time, and by age, sex, and numerous risk factors (Brody & Chen, 1969; Stanhope et al, 1972; Reed & Brody, 1975). Furthermore, there have been several genetic studies; but despite the conclusion stated in one report (Plato et al, 1969), no specific genetic pattern has been established and an exogenous cause appears far more likely to me. That view is supported by the recent report of 27 Chamorro marriages in which both spouses had either ALS or PD but no strong genetic trend was noted in the offspring of this presumably very high-risk group (Reed et al, 1975).

However, in spite of a considerable number of studies on the aetiology of ALS and PD on Guam, including the recent well designed case control effort by Reed et al (Reed & Brody, 1975; Reed et al, 1975), no specific agent has been identified.

The combination of prevalent neurological disease, collagen changes in the skin of the same patients, and the high incidence of dyschondroplasia (multiple exostoses) (Krooth et al, 1961) observed on Guam led to intensive efforts to find some local food with lathyrogenic properties. One source of such toxin that has aroused considerable interest is the nut of *Cycas circinalis* (cycad), which apparently has been an important food on the island for an uncertain but probably very long period (Kurland, 1972).

In their natural form, cycads may contain a small quantity of lathyrogenic substance that conceivably could affect motor and other neurones. However, about 5% of the Marianas cycad is a remarkable water-soluble hepatotoxic and carcinogenic agent, cycasin, which can be removed by thorough elution. Several species of animals have been tested with the aglycone of cycasin (methylazoxymethanol or MAM), which biochemically resembles dimethylnitrosamine. In large quantities, cycasin causes hepatic necrosis and rapid death and in smaller quantities, cirrhosis, and in minute quantities, it has produced hepatic and other tumours after a latent period of one year or more (Sixth International Cycad Conference in Federation Proceedings, 1972).

It is conceivable that, in the Marianas patients, minute quantities of cycasin could be retained because of inadequate washing of the nut and could lead to a hepatic disturbance in the production of some enzyme that is essential for the metabolism of motor neurones. Injection of cycasin or MAM in very young animals has induced cerebellar degeneration and reduced cerebral mass, but no specific motor neurone disease has been observed (Haddad et al, 1972; Hirono, 1972; Hirano & Jones, 1972; Jones et al, 1972). There remains the need to develop an appropriate animal model which might respond with motor degeneration (Mettler, 1972; Andrews & Andrews, 1976).

The pattern of use, many years ago, of prepared cycad flour that may have retained minute quantities of cycasin would be exceedingly difficult to demonstrate today. Cycad was prepared by families who harvested the nuts in the tropical forests and were expected to treat them by a ritual 7-day elution process before using the washed nuts as flour for food or barter. Occasional periods of lack of rain or an inadequate supply of treated cycad may have led to premature use. To further complicate the situation, unwashed cycad was said to have been used by the local herbalists as a poultice for the treatment of ulcers and other skin ailments; and in experiments, cycasin has been absorbed by animals under similar circumstances (O'Gara et al, 1964). The period between exposure to cycad and the development of ALS, if these are associated, might vary with the food preparation and health practices in the villages. The association with cycad may also be spurious if some fungal agent such as an aflatoxin contaminated the cycad occasionally in the soaking process. Such a relationship might be with certain lots of cycad which at this later date cannot be identified or traced.

If the recently observed decrease in the incidence of ALS and PD on Guam continues (Reed & Brody, 1975), it will correspond to the decrease in use of cycad. Before and during World War II, cycad was said to be the major source of carbohydrate for the entire native population of Guam. After 1945 it was replaced gradually by wheat, rice, and corn products with the westernisation of the local economy and diet as Guam became a major military centre and a supply centre for the US Trust Territories. But the westernisation of Guam in recent years has produced many other dramatic changes in living patterns, and some element other than cycad usage could be responsible for the decreasing incidence of ALS and PD.

The possible influences of infection, other nutritional agents, and heavy metals are still being explored. Manganese, calcium, and parathyroid hormone are being considered by the team at Wakayama University, which is investigating ALS in the Kii Peninsula (Yase et al, 1974).

After the observation that C-type virus was present in wild mice in California that developed a motor neurone disease (Andrews & Garner, 1974), a search was initiated for C-type particles in the brains and spinal cords of Guamanian patients, but no conclusive results with respect to ALS have been obtained (Brody, 1976).

The case control comparison on Guam was developed with a standardised interview of ALS or PD cases and randomly chosen controls. The comparison did not reveal any patterns of prior illness, life style, or exposure differentiating patients and controls. The patients tended to be of somewhat lower socioeconomic level, had less education, ate more homegrown foods and raw meat, and had greater contact with animals. A very high percentage of cases and controls reported previous use of cycad (Reed & Brody, 1975; Reed et al, 1975).

Some familial aggregation among cases was noted, but no mendelian genetic patterns were observed. The authors concluded: "It is possible that genetic influences affect the occurrence of these diseases but our studies suggest that environmental factors play at least as important a role" (Reed et al, 1975) . . . . "Environmental factors associated with some aspect of the traditional way of life seem to be causally involved but, since most aspects of the traditional life have changed in the past 50 years, the specific factors remain elusive" (Reed & Brody, 1975).

Sporadic Form

Almost every mechanism that seems plausible has been considered at some time in the search for the cause of sporadic ALS, and this review will not touch upon all of them. A few items of special interest will be mentioned, but the emphasis will be on reported or ongoing case control comparisons.

An infectious aetiology has been pursued for many years. Zil'ber and associates in the USSR reported transmission of ALS to laboratory primates in 1961 (Zil'ber, 1961), but the changes could not be verified by several veterinary neuropathologists in whose company I visited the Soviet Union for a scientific exchange programme in 1964 (Brody et al, 1965). Gibbs and Gajdusek, using techniques identical to those that were successful for kuru, have inoculated chimpanzees, other primates, and animals of other orders and have tried numerous routine diagnostic laboratory tests for more than 10 years, but have so far failed to detect the presence of a virus (Gibbs & Gajdusek, 1972). Cremer et al (1973) were also unable to obtain a viral clue of the disease through cell cultures or serum antibody titres. Using lymphocyte transformation with patients and controls and brain material from ALS and PD patients and controls, Chen et al (1970) could find no evidence that hyperimmune mechanisms were involved.

In studies of ALS patients and controls at the University of Mississippi Hospital, ALS seemed to have a predilection for persons who did heavy labour, including farmers (Breland & Currier, 1967). Heavy metals have been considered from time to time in the aetiology of ALS, but the amount of lead and mercury found in tissues of the Mississippi patients as a group was not greater than normal (Currier & Haerer, 1968). Pyruvate levels in their blood and spinal fluid were normal also, and this was interpreted as ruling out acute arsenic or recent heavy-metal intoxication.

In their recent case control study Felmus et al (1976) inquired about a large number of suspected risk factors in 25 patients and 50 controls. Their report implies that there were significant differences with respect to reported exposure to lead and mercury, participation in athletics, and consumption of large quantities of milk. Some question might be raised about the appropriateness of the controls (25 were patients with other neurological diseases and the rest were hospital employees). Unfortunately, a more serious criticism is that an inappropriate method of statistical testing was used, which resulted in induly small and probably erroneous P values that were interpreted as statistically significant.

In an ongoing study by Mulder and Kurland, comparison of findings in 68 patients and 68 controls (unaffected sibling, spouse, or friend of the patient) provided no substantiation of the differences reported by Felmus et al.

Henderson at the University of Southern California also has a large case control study under way, but so far has found no significantly elevated risk ratio for rural place of birth, foreign travel, previous medical history, outdoor activities, or the consumption of sheep or calf brain (Henderson, 1976).

The most rigorous series of current studies is being made through the US Veterans' Administration under the auspices of the Follow-Up Agency of the National Research Council (Beebe, 1976). It is an epidemiological survey of the military records of World War II veterans with ALS and controls who died from 1963 through 1967; and there are plans to conduct an intensive interview inquiry of a large number of patients and controls in Veterans' Administration hospitals. Results are not yet available, and scepticism remains that in this type of investigation the right questions may not be asked and the effort will fail to ferret out those antecedent events that are associated with the disease. We may hope that, if these inquiries are not successful, further studies will benefit from the experience acquired or it may be necessary to await some breakthrough in the laboratories.

SUMMARY AND CONCLUSIONS

In the past two decades, the epidemiological approach to amyotrophic lateral sclerosis has provided considerable information on the incidence, geographical patterns, and population selectivity of the disorder. Knowledge of the geographical pattern (particularly the foci of ALS in the Western Pacific Islands) and of familial aggregation of cases has led to the conclusion that there are at least three major types of ALS, which are referred to as (1) sporadic, (2) familial and presumably hereditary, and (3) Western Pacific or Marianas form. Studied aimed at clarifying the aetiology of ALS should consider the great likelihood that the causes of these forms differ.

With considerable information of a descriptive nature on ALS now available, the increased use of case control comparisons in different localities seems timely and appropriate, even though results to date may be more controversial than enlightening. Review of the methods of such comparisons emphasises the advantages of matching controls in some instances and selecting randomly from the population in others.

Presumably, ALS is due to a combination of genetically determined and exogenous factors. The familial form is probably metabolic in origin, with exogenous factors exerting a minimal influence in precipitating the onset of disease. In each of the other two forms, there is presumably some inherent predisposition, but an exogenous factor is probably of appreciable importance. The specific agents are unknown, though in the Marianas type it may be cycad-related. If that proves to be so, some azoxy or nitrosamine-like agent may be among factors causing the sporadic form in other parts of the world. A breakthrough in the aetiology of any one form should facilitate the recognition of causes and could lead to control of the other forms of ALS as well.

References

Alpert, JN, Stevens, PM, Levine, CP (1972) *Clinical and Autopsy Report No N-72-226, Methodist Hospital, Houston, Texas.* Unpublished data

Anderson, FH, Richardson, EP Jr, Okazaki, H and Brody, JA (1976) *Alzheimer's neurofibrillary changes on Guam: Frequency in Chamorros and non Chamorros with no known neurological disease.* Unpublished data

Andrews, JM and Andrews, RL (1976) *The comparative neuropathology of motor neuron diseases.* Unpublished data

Andrews, GM and Garner, MB (1974) *Neurology (Minneap), 24,* 383

Arnason, B (1976) Personal communication

Bebbe, G (1976) Personal communication

Bobowick, AR and Brody, JA (1973) *New England Journal of Medicine, 288,* 1047

Breland, AE, and Currier, RD (1967) *Neurology (Minneap), 17,* 1011

Brody, J (1976) Personal communication

Brody, JA and Chen, KM (1969) In *Motor Neuron Diseases.* (Ed) FH Norris Jr and LT Kurland. Grune & Stratton, New York. Page 61

Brody, JA and Kurland, LT (1973) In *Tropical Neurology.* (Ed) JD Spillane. Oxford University Press, Oxford. Page 355

Brody, JA et al (1965) *Science, 147,* 1114

Chen, KM, Brody, JA, Kurland, LT and Elizan, TS (1970) *Neurology (Minneap), 20,* 954

Colton, T (1974) *Statistics in Medicine.* Little, Brown and Company, New York

Cremer, NE, Oshiro, LS, Norris, FH, Lennette, EH (1973) *Archives of Neurology, 29,* 331

Currier, RD, Haerer, AF (1968) *Archives of Environmental Health, 17,* 712

Engel, K, Kurland, LT and Klatzo, I (1959) *Brain, 82,* 203

Felmus, MT, Patten, BM and Swanke, L (1976) *Neurology (Minneap), 26,* 167

Fullmer, HM, Diedler, HD, Krooth, RS and Kurland, LT (1960) *Neurology (Minneap), 10,* 717

Gibbs, CJ, Gajdusek, DC (1972) *Parkinson's Disease, and the amyotrophic lateral sclerosis-Parkinsonism-demential Complex on Guam: A Review and Summary of attempts to demonstrate infection as the aetiology. Royal College of Pathologists – Host-Virus Reactions, symposium supplement.* Page 132

Haddad, RK, Rabe, A and Dumas, R (1972) *Federation Proceedings, 31,* 1520

Henderson, B (1976) Personal communication

Hirano, A and Jones, M (1972) *Federation Proceedings, 31,* 1517

Hirano, A, Kurland, LT, Krooth, RS and Lessell, S (1961) *Brain, 84,* 642

Hirano, A, Malamud, N and Kurland, LT (1961) *Brain, 84,* 662

Hirano, A, Malamud, N, Kurland, LT and Zimmerman, HM (1969) In *Motor Neuron Diseases.* (Ed) FH Norris Jr and LT Kurland. Grune & Stratton, New York. Page 51

Hirono, I (1972) *Federation Proceedings, 31,* 1493

Jones, J, Yang, M and Mickelsen, O (1972) *Federation Proceedings, 31,* 1508

Kimura, K et al (1963) *Diseases of the Nervous System, 24,* 155

Krooth, RS, Macklin, MT and Hillbish, TF (1961) *American Journal of Human Genetics, 13,* 340

Kurland, LT (1972) *Federation Proceedings, 31,* 1540

Kurland, LT and Brody, JA (1975) In *The Nervous System. Volume 2: The Clinical Neurosciences.* (Editor-in-Chief) DB Tower. Raven Press, New York

Kurland, LT and Mulder, DW (1954) *Neurology (Minneap), 4, No 5-6*
Kurland, LT and Mulder, DW (1955) *Neurology (Minneap), 5,* 182 and 249
Kurland, LT, Kurtzke, JF and Goldberg, ID (1973) In *Epidemiology of Neurologic and Sense Organ Disorders. Vital and Health Statistics Monographs, American Public Health Association.* Harvard University Press. Page 108
Kurland, LT, Won Choi, N and Sayre, GP (1969) In *Motor Neuron Diseases.* (Ed) FH Norris Jr and LT Kurland. Grune & Stratton, New York. Page 28
Matsumoto, N, Worth, RM, Kurland, LT and Okazaki, I (1972) *Neurology (Minneap), 22,* 934
Mettler, FA (1972) *Federation Proceedings, 31,* 1504
Norris, F (1974) *Recent Advances in Motor Neuron Diseases. International Congress Series No 360.* Excerpta Medica, Amsterdam
Norris, F (1976) *Diagnostic and Prognostic profiles in amyotrophic lateral sclerosis.* Unpublished data
Norris, FH Jr, McMenemey, WH and Barnard, RO (1969) In *Motor Neuron Diseases.* (Ed) FH Norris Jr and LT Kurland. Grune & Stratton, New York. Page 100
O'Gara, RW, Brown, JM and Whiting, MG (1964) *Federation Proceedings, 23,* 1383
Oldstone, MBA, Wilson, CB and Dalessio, D (1973) *Transactions of the American Neurological Association, 98,* 181
Plato, CC, Cruz, MT and Kurland, LT (1969) *American Journal of Human Genetics, 21,* 133
Reed, DM and Brody, JA (1975) *American Journal of Epidemiology, 101,* 287
Reed, D, Plato, C, Elizan, T and Kurland, LT (1966) *American Journal of Epidemiology, 83,* 54
Reed, DM, Torres, JM and Brody, JA (1975) *American Journal of Epidemiology, 101,* 302
Shiraki, Y and Yase, Y (1975) In *The Handbook of Clinical Neurology.* (Ed) P Vinken and G Bruyn. North Holland Publishing Co, Amsterdam
Sixth International Cycad Conference (1972) In *Federation Proceedings (Federation of American Societies for Experimental Biology)* Sept—Oct
Stanhope, JM, Brody, JA and Morris, CE (1972) *International Journal of Epidemiology, 1,* 199
Yase, Y, Matsumoto, N, Yoshimasu, F, Handa, Y and Kumamoto, T (1968) *Proceedings of the Australian Association of Neurology, 5,* 335
Yase, Y, Yoshimasu, F, Uebayashi, Y, Iwata, S and Kumura, K (1974) *Proceedings of the Japanese Academy, 50,* 401
Zil'ber, LA (1961) *Bulletin of the World Health Organisation, 29* 449

CHAPTER THREE

ABIOTROPHY REVISITED

P D Lewis

For the physician, the validity of observation is generally greater than that of hypothesis - but "there is a region in which we must recognise hypothesis as absolute. It is the region below the surface whence no reflected light can pass, but whence all observed phenomena proceed. Here we must accept indirect perception, or we must be content with no perception of the causes of that we observe".

William Gowers, in his 1894 lecture on 'Dynamics of life', was discussing what was known of muscle and nerve physiology at the time. Although he was able to analyse the manifestations of energy in movement and sensation, he could not envisage the relation of energy to life, and implied that this relationship, and the nature of the life-force itself, could never be understood. This mystical attitude, which is central to Gowers' concept of abiotrophy, was not unique to the famous neurologist. It was current in the last years of the nineteenth century, and in his lecture Gowers was echoing amongst others Samuel Butler, who was preoccupied with the synthesis of mechanistic and metaphysical, and whose 'Erewhon revisited' I quite unconsciously echoed in my title. Thus abiotrophy, discussed fully by Gowers in 1902, has a mystical core, the nature of life, a life that is perceived indirectly, by negative staining, through the effects of its departure from nerve cells and muscle fibres.

While medical Greek or Latin, applied to an obscure syndrome, is generally less valuable (since less honest) than the straightforward expression of ignorance conveyed by an eponym, Gowers' invention remains useful today. There is no other simple expression, as he wrote, to designate the concept of "a degeneration or decay in consequence of a defect of vital endurance"; and if we demystify it by concentrating on the nature of the intrinsic defect responsible, rather than that of life itself, we may stand to gain some understanding of such disorders as motor neurone disease (MND).

The intrinsic defect in motor cells in MND is of course still quite unknown, and advance in understanding is hampered by the lack of an obvious experimental model. But if, like Gowers, we accept "indirect perception" the problem can be approached in the laboratory. For there are other types and patterns of nerve cell death, and here the "defects of vital endurance" are amenable to experiment. These fall into the category of physiological cell death, and I propose to review what is known about the mechanism of physiological cell death in the nervous system. I hope that its analysis may ultimately cast light on the processes involved in MND, and perhaps eventually allow us to modify its course. Avenues of research into this terrible disease are few, and this is surely one worth following. My thesis is this: first, that the lethal sequence of events which ends in nerve cell death in MND may have features in common with what happens in some cells in the normal nervous system at the two extremes of a lifespan; and secondly, that this occurrence, 'physiological cell death', which is open to laboratory investigation, may constitute a valid model for MND.

The term 'physiological cell death' is used to cover a number of phenomena that have been discovered in such widely separated fields as embryology, ageing research, and experimental pathology. These include the destruction of large numbers of cells, often in well defined populations such as the anterior horns of the spinal cord, at specific points during development; loss of cells in ageing organs, both sporadically and in major episodes; and shrinkage, fragmentation and lysis of cells in response to essentially non-pathological stimuli, such as hormones. A factor common to these forms of cell death, and to abiotrophy in the strict sense, is an absence of any identifiable exogenous influence, toxic or infective, or a recognisable, externally correctible deficiency state.

This is a large field of research activity, and a great deal of information is available (Glücksmann, 1951; Lockshin & Beaulaton, 1974). Yet cell death is still a somewhat unfamiliar topic, even to the point of not having a discoverable entry of its own in the Cumulative Index Medicus. The reasons for this unfamiliarity are unclear. One can speculate on its relation to the prevailing attitude to death in our society, or even to a false image of ageing research as the province of charlatans and eccentrics. However the strangeness of the concept of cell death is surely tied up with the widely held belief, first expressed by Alexis Carrell in 1912, that cells had a permanent life, an immortality, when maintained under optimal conditions in culture outside the body. If individual cells were indeed potentially immortal, then their death from endogenous causes was to be expected when the body died, but hardly otherwise, except perhaps in senescence; so cell death as a physiological phenomenon occurring at other periods of life could have little meaning. Neither could abiotrophy, or selective cell death due to comparable phenomena, make any scientific sense.

It was only in 1961 that the immortality of normal diploid cells in culture (as distinct from neoplastic cells) was shown to be a myth. Hayflick & Moorhead cultured normal human fibroblasts derived from foetal lung tissue. After a period of active multiplication in culture, cells took longer to divide, gradually lost their mitotic activity, accumulated debris and ultimately died. It was shown that a population of fibroblasts was only capable of about 50 doublings, over a period of about six months. Subsequently, after repeated confirmation of this finding, fibroblast clones derived from single cells isolated from mass cultures were studied by Smith & Hayflick (1974). These had variable life spans, but the greatest doubling potential in a clone was about the same as that of the mass culture from which the parent cell had been obtained. Thus a limited capacity to divide appears to be an innate feature of all cells cultured in vitro. This limit varies with the species, and is lower in chicken and mice, which have a relatively short life span, than in man (Lima and Macieira-Coelho, 1972; Todaro & Green, 1963). Survival also decreases with increasing age of the donor: Martin et al (1970) cultured skin fibroblasts from the forearm of donors ranging from infancy to 90, and found that the average rate of decrease was 0.2 population doublings per year of donor life. In subjects with Werner's syndrome fibroblasts were capable of only 25% or less of the number of population doublings expected on the basis of the donor's age.

Cell death of mass cultures in Hayflick's phase III, analogous to the Go phase of the generative cycle of individual dividing cells, must be interpreted as an inevitable consequence of underlying, non-disease-related biological events. Before discussing the possible nature of these changes, it is worth noting that the vast majority of nerve cells are in their postmitotic non-dividing (Go) phase for the entire postnatal lifespan. They would thus be ideal candidates for those changes that might be responsible for death of aged cells in tissue culture. The question of 'cell loss with age among fixed postmitotics' (Comfort, 1971) is still incompletely answered, but such careful studies as those of Hall et al (1975) confirm that decline in numbers in a nerve cell population occurs with advancing age (in this case, over 60 years). These authors counted human cerebellar Purkinje cells, but we do not as yet know for sure whether comparable cell loss occurs in the cerebral cortex or anterior horns of the spinal cord — and therefore whether clinical symptoms and signs can be related to such a process. However, it may well be fallacious to regard healthy nerve cells as immortal. Their death in old age could be seen as an inevitable event, the consequence of a cumulatively lethal series of molecular defects, rather than as the chance result of damage by hypoxia or an infective agent, deficiency or intoxication. This series of molecular defects could also operate in the exaggerated and premature cell death of MND, and in the cell death which is such a prominent feature in the developing nervous system. It is known that in the normal chick, only about 60% of the motor neurones laid down in the lateral column of the lumbar spinal cord survive through the development period, while in the mouse even fewer may remain (Hamburger, 1975; Flanagan, 1969). In the chick, the deficient fraction of the motor neurones degenerate between 6 and 9 days of embryonic life, and in the mouse between fetal days 11 and 14. The loss occurs at a time when the muscles have developed and are being innervated. It is thus related to the establishment of provisional nerve contact with muscle fibres, and may well be a consequence on the one hand of over-production of neurones at an earlier stage, when the quantitative requirements at the periphery cannot be accurately anticipated, and on the other, of competition for receptor sites, the recognition of which involves a degree of trial and error. However, these and other occurrences of degeneration in the developing nervous system (see for example Romanes, 1946; Hamburger & Levi-Montalcini, 1949; Lewis, 1975; Lewis et al, 1976) may well have a common basis which is ultimately centrally rather than peripherally determined.

Those cells which die can be shown to be postmitotic, and have possibly been withdrawn from the proliferative pool. Further, it is likely that in these, as in other doomed embryonic cells, morphological evidence of cell death is preceded by a decrease in protein synthesis (Pollak & Fallon, 1974). The molecular lesion behind these events is obscure, but in a situation which is highly amenable to experiment, with evolution of events over a short, rather than protracted time period, and with the possibility of separating neuronal populations and increasing the amount of cell death occurring in it by such a simple measure as undernutrition (Balàzs et al, 1974; Lewis, 1975), investigation is mandatory. Are the underlying events the same as those implicated in normal ageing? And are these events responsible too for cell death in MND?

These questions take us back to ageing research, and I shall conclude by introducing the theory of somatic mutation into this discussion of the molecular mechanisms implicated in cell death. As first formulated, this theory ascribed the ageing process to progressive accumulation of gene mutations in somatic cells. However, the indirectly calculated mutation rate is too low to account for gross impairment of cell function during the lifetime of an individual, and the theory has had to be modified. Gene mutation would have the effect of causing synthesis of abnormal messenger RNA and in turn faulty proteins; current theory (Orgel, 1963), focusing on the formation of faulty proteins, ascribes this not to gene mutation but to impaired specificity of the enzymes involved in the translation mechanisms. The concept of 'error-catastrophe' describes the situation in which errors due to impaired specificity of information-handling enzymes in protein synthesis lead to an increasing error frequency, building up to the point at which a metabolic process necessary for the viability of the cell becomes critically inefficient. The theory predicts that the introduction of incorrect aminoacids would accelerate ageing and cell death, and that increasing amounts of non-functional protein would be detectable in ageing cells. Such predictions have been confirmed experimentally (Holliday, 1969; Lewis & Holliday, 1970).

Changes in the information content of DNA might well contribute to 'error-catastrophe'. How these might come about is unknown. Repair of DNA could be faulty in those cells destined to die. Recently, the severity of neurological abnormality in patients with xeroderma pigmentosum has been found to be related to the patients' ability to repair ultraviolet-induced DNA damage (Andrews et al, 1976). Patients with the most severe neurological abnormalities (allegedly due to premature nerve cell death, and including lower motor neurone involvement, but without autopsy confirmation of anterior horn cell loss: see Robbins et al, 1974) had the least effective DNA repair, as shown by decreased colony-forming ability on the part of UV-irradiated fibroblasts. The authors suggested that the lack of adequate DNA repair was causally related to the clinical manifestations of a human 'degenerative' neurological disease, implicating Orgel's error-catastrophe hypothesis. This suggestion may be premature, but is worth noting as indicating an area of future study. Another line of thought implicates 5-methyl cytosine, an obligatory minor component of animal DNA which is believed to be involved in cellular differentiation (Scarano et al, 1967). One report suggests that this base is present in the DNA of brain cells in relatively high concentration compared with other organs, though not in old animals, where the concentration in different organs is uniform (Vanyushin et al, 1973). If this finding is confirmed, could the progressive elimination of this base with age be implicated in nerve cell death through the mechanisms already outlined?

I have tried to indicate some ways in which a combination of biochemical and morphological approaches, perhaps applied to the developing nervous system, may throw some light on the mechanism of neuronal death. Valid models of motor neurone disease may already be staring us in the face, and the disease may not be as mystical and mysterious as we think. Once the mechanisms of cell death have been defined, we may be in a position to modify them.

References

Andrews, AD, Barrett, SF and Robbins, JH (1976) *Lancet, i,* 1318
Balàzs, R, Hajós, F, Johnson, AL, Tapia, R and Wilkin, G (1974) *Biochemical Society Transactions, 2,* 682
Carrell, A (1912) *Journal of Experimental Medicine, 15,* 516
Comfort, A (1971) *Nature, 229,* 282
Flanagan, AEH (1969) *Journal of Morphology, 129,* 281
Glücksmann, A (1951) *Biological Reviews, 26,* 59
Gowers, WR (1894) *Dynamics of Life.* Churchill, London
Gowers, WR (1902) *Lancet, i,* 1003
Hall, TC, Miller, AKH and Corsellis, JAN (1975) *Neuropathology and Applied Neurobiology, 1,* 267
Hamburger, V (1975) *Journal of Comparative Neurology, 160,* 535
Hamburger, V and Levi-Montalcini, R (1949) *Journal of Experimental Zoology, 111,* 457
Hayflick, L and Moorhead, PS (1961) *Experimental Cell Research, 25,* 585
Holliday, R (1969) *Nature, 221,* 1224
Lewis, CM and Holliday, R (1970) *Nature, 228,* 877
Lewis, PD (1975) *Neuropathology and Applied Neurobiology, 1,* 21
Lewis, PD, Patel, AJ, Johnson, AL and Balazs, R (1976) *Brain Research, 104,* 49

Lima, L and Macieira-Coelho, A (1972) *Experimental Cell Research, 70,* 279

Lockshin, RA and Beaulaton, J (1974) *Life Sciences, 15,* 1549

Martin, GM, Sprague, CA and Epstein, CJ (1970) *Laboratory Investigation, 23,* 86

Orgel, LE (1963) *Proceedings of the National Academy of Sciences of the United States of America, 49,* 517

Pollak, RD and Fallon, JF (1974) *Experimental Cell Research, 84,* 9

Robbins, JH, Kraemer, KH, Lutzner, MA, Festoff, BW and Coon, HG (1974) *Annals of Internal Medicine, 80,* 221

Romanes, GJ (1946) *Journal of Anatomy (London), 80,* 117

Scarano, E, Iaccarino, M, Grippo, P and Parisi, E (1967) *Proceedings of the National Academy of Sciences of the United States of America, 57,* 1394

Smith, JR and Hayflick, L (1974) *Journal of Cell Biology, 62,* 48

Todaro, GJ and Green, H (1963) *Journal of Cell Biology, 17,* 299

Vanuyshin, BF, Mazin, AL, Vasilyev, VK and Belozersky, AN (1973) *Biochimica et Biophysica Acta, 299,* 397

CHAPTER FOUR

AXONAL TRANSPORT AND ITS POSSIBLE ROLE
IN MOTOR NEURONE DISEASE

W G Bradley

This chapter reviews axonal transport and speculates on its role in the aetiology of motor neurone disease. Since the earliest days of histology it has been known that the neurones have a large amount of basophilic material in the cell body. More recently this has been shown to be due to masses of rough endoplasmic reticulum which are responsible for the high rate of protein synthesis of neurones. From the beginning of the microscopy of living cells in vitro, movement of particles within these cells has been recognised, particularly in neurones (Nakai, 1964; Allen, 1967; Breuer et al, 1975). The last 30 years have seen the gradual accumulation of the knowledge required to explain these observations.

Particles within neurones in tissue culture move at up to 9 um per second, which is equivalent to 780 mm/day, and is similar to the rate of movement seen in other cells (Jahn and Bovee, 1969; Rebhun, 1972). Under direct observation particles may be seen moving in both orthograde and retrograde directions, starting and stopping, and changing directions. The outgrowing tip of neurones in tissue culture grow at about 1–2 mm/day (Nakai, 1964), and regeneration of nerves in vivo proceeds at an approximately similar rate (Sunderland, 1968).

Methods of the Study of Axonal Transport

1. The direct visualisation of the movement of particles within axons   This has been undertaken in neurones in vitro by many workers (Nakai, 1964), and has been used in excised peripheral axons in vitro using Nomarski microscopy (Kirkpatrick et al, 1972). Unfortunately it is only useful for the study of the movement of particles, and not that of soluble substances, and is difficult to quantitate (Breuer et al, 1975).

36

2. Ligation experiments   A ligature applied around a nerve will block all transport across the ligated zone. Provided the study is conducted for only a short period, and the accumulation of material above the ligature is linear for that period, then the rate of transport and the amount of material moving may be determined.

At time *t* after ligation, if E units of the substance under study are present in a segment L mm long immediately above the ligature, and C units are present in the comparable segment L mm long in the opposite non-ligated nerve, then the rate of axonal transport of the substance is given by the equation:

$$\text{Rate} = \frac{E - C}{C} \times \frac{L}{t} \text{ mm/hr}$$

$$\text{and Amount} = \text{Rate} \times \frac{C}{L} \text{ units/hr}$$

It is better to derive the rate of accumulation of material from the slope of the line relating accumulation to time. These estimates assume that all the substance is mobile but it is quite likely that this assumption is not correct, in which case the estimates of rate are too low, and of amount are too high. Moreover the technique is not strictly physiological since the ligation blocks retrograde axonal transport, and local changes at the site of ligation and alterations to the cyton function may be caused by ligation. Another difficulty with this technique is that it is only able to determine one rate of transport; a second rate would be shown as non-linearity of the rate of accumulation, and would be difficult to interpret. Nevertheless nerve ligation studies are relatively easy and quick to perform, and have revealed useful results.

3. Pulse-labelling experiments of the cyton   Radioactive-labelled amino acid administered to an animal labels the protein, first within the neurone cyton in relation to the Nissl substance, and later some of this protein is exported down the axon (Droz and LeBlond, 1963). No labelled protein is seen in the main axon until it arrives from the cyton, correlating with the absence of significant amounts of RNA in mammalian axons, and necessitating that all the proteins of the axon are synthesised within the cyton. This probably explains the breakdown of the peripheral axon following section (Wallerian degeneration). The situation is different in giant axons such as those of the squid, and in nerves of amphibia, where protein synthetic machinery is present within the axons, which can therefore survive for long periods after separation from the cyton.

Labelled material is not all exported from the cyton at the same time as much remains static within the cell body. The labelled material which reaches the axon travels at different rates and, once it reaches the axon, transport is independent of the cyton, continuing after separation from the cell body.

Two major rates of the flow of proteins have been described in such pulse-labelling experiments; a slow flow of 1–5 mm/day, and a fast flow of about 400 mm/day. These values are interestingly similar to the polar values for particle movement and nerve growth described above. Though some have suggested that slow (Weiss, 1972) or fast (Ochs, 1974a) are the only rates of axonal flow, it is clear that there are many intermediate rates (Bradley et al, 1971; Karlsson and Sjöstrand, 1971 a and b). The relative amounts of material moving at the different rates vary in different systems but, where the overall flow of protein has been studied, the material transported at slow rates exceeds the amount transported at fast by about one order of magnitude.

Quantitation of the amount of material transported at different rates is possible in pulse-labelling experiments such as shown in Figure 1. The rate of movement may either be determined from the front or the crest of the wave, and the amount by the height of the crest. Due to difficulties in ensuring that

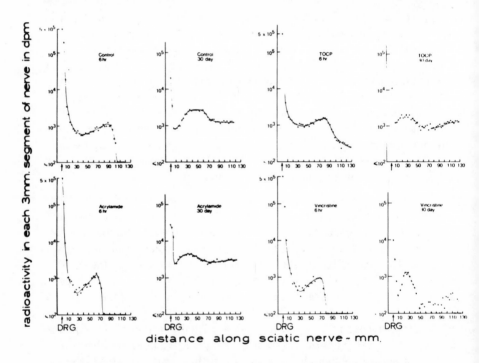

Figure 1 Distribution of radioactivity in 3 mm segments of L7 dorsal root ganglia and sciatic nerves of cats 6 hr and 30 days after injection of ³H-leucine into the dorsal root ganglia. Each point is the average of values from 3 animals. Control animals, and those intoxicated with acrylamide. triorthocresyl phosphate and vincristine are shown (after Bradley and Williams, 1973)

the same dose of labelled amino acid precursor is given to different animals, it is usual to normalise the data by expressing the radioactive level of the crest as a ratio of the radioactive level of the cyton. Thus in the study of Bradley and Williams (1973 − Figure 1) the average rate of movement of the fast component in control cats was 459 mm/day for the front and 385mm/day for the crest of the wave, with an average crest/ganglion level of 0.47%. For the slow component, the average rate of movement of the crest was 1.4 mm/day, with a crest/ganglion level of 12.6%.

Further studies have demonstrated many different substances moving in an orthograde fashion by axonal transport, including individual protein species, enzymes and neurotubular protein (Grafstein et al, 1970), glycoproteins, catecholamines, mitochondria and probably RNA and phospholipids. Moreover some substances move in a relatively limited velocity band; for instance glycoproteins are rapidly transported (Forman et al, 1971, 1972; Edström and Mattson, 1972); mitochondria move at fast rates (Jeffrey and Austin, 1973); choline acetyltransferase is transported at a slower rate than acetylcholinesterase (Tuček, 1975). Subcellular fractionation studies of the localisation of proteins at different periods after the injection of a radioactive-labelled amino acid precursor indicate that though most of the protein is in the soluble fraction at all times, at the earliest times corresponding to the fastest rates, there is a significantly higher specific activity in the particulate fraction (McEwen and Grafstein, 1968; Kidwai and Ochs, 1969; Sjöstrand and Karlsson, 1969; Sjöstrand, 1970).

Axonal transport has been shown to depend upon the supply of energy (Ochs and Ranish, 1970; Ochs, 1974b), on the temperature (Grafstein et al, 1972; Ochs and Smith, 1975); on the integrity of the neurotubules (Barondes, 1967; Schmitt and Samson, 1968), being blocked by substances causing depolymerisation of neurotubules such as colchicine, vincristine and vinblastine (inter al Karlsson and Sjöstrand, 1969; James et al, 1970a; Sjöstrand et al, 1970; Fink et al, 1973; Frizzell et al, 1975) or those stabilising neurotubules such as heavy water (Anderson et al, 1972). Axonal transport may depend on the integrity of microfilaments since cytochalasin B impairs axonal transport (Crooks and McClure, 1972; Fernandez and Samson, 1973; McGregor et al, 1973). Axonal transport occurs both in myelinated and unmyelinated fibres, though the amount and rate are somewhat more in unmyelinated fibres (Sjöstrand, 1970; Ochs and Jersild, 1974; Gross and Beidler, 1975; Somerville and Bradley, 1976).

Repeated stimulation of a neurone increases the rate of axonal transport (Jasinski et al, 1966; Kreutzberg and Schubert, 1973), though axonal transport in the optic nerves of rabbits reared in the dark is similar to those reared in the light (Karlsson and Sjöstrand, 1971c). However, axonal transport is not dependent on nerve action potentials since it continues despite blockage of the axolemmal sodium channels by tetrodotoxin (Ochs and Hollingsworth, 1971), and despite major alterations of the extracellular ion concentrations (Edström, 1975). Increase of the intracellular sodium concentration by batrachotoxin, however, blocks fast axonal transport (Ochs and Worth, 1975). Local anaesthetics in low concentration, while blocking the nerve action potential, probably have no effect on axonal transport but lignocaine and other local anaesthetics in higher concentrations do block axonal transport (Fink et al, 1972; Bisby, 1975). General anaesthetics also probably have no effect on axonal transport (Fink and Kennedy, 1972). Axonal transport is faster in developing nerves (Bondy and Madsen, 1971; Marchisio et al, 1973), but in regenerating nerves the transport of some substances is increased and that of others decreased (Frizzell and Sjöstrand, 1974).

4. Retrograde transport   That particles move in a retrograde direction has been known for many years from direct microscopic observation of nerves. Tetanus toxin and rabies virus are believed to invade the central nervous system by retrograde movement along axons. More recently, retrograde axonal transport has been clearly demonstrated by the peripheral injection of amino acids and tracer proteins like horseradish peroxidase and Evans blue-albumin, studying the rate of accumulation of these substances within the cyton (Watson, 1968; Kristensson and Olsson, 1973; Bunt et al, 1974). Retrograde transport has also been studied by measuring the accumulation of substances below a ligature on a nerve. From such studies it is clear that the rate and mount of retrograde transport is less than the orthograde, though there is less quantitative data concerning retrograde transport than orthograde. Though the retrograde transport of certain substances like nerve growth factor has a molecular specificity (Hendry et al, 1974; Stoeckel et al, 1975), that of horseradish peroxidase and similar substances is probably non-specific.

The Mechanism of Axonal Transport

A variety of theories of axonal transport have been propounded since the phenomenon was first recognised. Weiss and Hiscoe (1948), who were responsible for the development of early concepts of axonal transport conceived of the mechanism of bulk synthesis by the cyton and secretion into the axon (Weiss, 1970). While this is probably true for regenerating nerves (which they were studying) or developing axons, it is unlikely to be the explanation in the mature state. Later Weiss and colleagues (Weiss, 1972; Biondi et al, 1972) concentrated on mechanical factors which might play a role, noting the contractions of Schwann cells and of axons seen in vitro, and suggesting axonal peristalsis as a possible mechanism for axonal transport. Cytoplasmic movement is however a feature of all cells, even plant cells with a rigid cellulose wall (Jahn and Bovee, 1969). It thus seems more likely that transport mechanisms relate to the internal structure of the cell.

With the demonstration that neurotubules were very much like the tubules of the mitotic spindle, cilia and flagella, and that the movement of the latter could be abolished by mitotic inhibitors such as colchicine and vinblastine, which also block axonal transport, the neurotubule theory was advanced (Barondes, 1967; Schmitt and Samson, 1968). The chemical structure of neuro-tubular protein (tubulin) is very similar to that of actin, with the association of a high energy phosphate compound, GTP. Myosin-like proteins have been isolated from the axon. On the basis of these observations, Schmitt (1968) suggested that substances move within the axons in a fashion similar to the sliding filament theory of muscle contraction, actin and myosin moving relative to one another by the repeated making and breaking, in the case of the nerve, of actin-GTP-myosin bonds with the interaction of calcium. Intraneural calcium has been shown to be necessary for axonal transport, though it appeared to act on the cyton rather than on the axon (Hammerschlag et al, 1975; Dravid and Hammer-schlag, 1975). Schmitt (1968) suggested that vesicles of myosin-like proteins might roll along neurotubules, a rolling or sliding vesicle theory.

Kerkut (1975) suggested a refinement of this, the coded vesicle theory in which the neurotubules were thought to act only as a cytoskeletal fixed phase. He suggested that actin filaments were tightly bound to the neurotubules, and that myosin molecules of various lengths occurred throughout the axoplasm. Substances to be moved at different rates within the axon were suggested to become encapsulated within vesicles, the outer coat of which had a specific code indicating the rate at which those vesicles were to be moved. This code was supposed to allow the vesicle to contact its appropriate myosin filament, the length of which was proportional to the speed of movement, larger ones with more side arms being supposed to move substances faster. Most myosin molecules were supposed to 'point' in an orthograde fashion, and the remainder in a retro-grade direction. Such a mechanism may underlie the faster rates of axonal trans-port where movement of the particulate fraction is particularly seen. However, the slower rates of transport are related mainly to soluble proteins, and the problem of both the rolling vesicle and the coded vesicle theories are that vesicles are relatively infrequently seen in the axoplasm under the electron microscope. It seems more likely that vesicles as such are not involved, and that substances to be transported can be linked, perhaps through carrier molecules, with myosin-like proteins, which can then be transported over the actin-like groups of the neurotubules. This might be termed the carrier molecule theory (Figure 2) and is an amplification of the transport filament theory of Ochs (1971, 1974a). Each substance would have a specific carrier; the direction of movement would be perhaps ordained by the orientation of myosin molecules as suggested by Kerkut (1975).

Gross (1975) suggested an alternative theory based on the neurotubules, the microstream theory, in which he suggested the presence of a zone of very low viscosity around the neurotubules, fading progressively with distance from the neurotubule into the highly viscous axoplasm. By combining this concept with

41

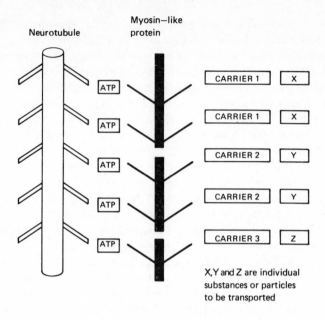

Figure 2 Schematic diagram of the carrier molecule theory of axonal transport. Individual substances to be transported might each be linked with myosin-like molecules via specific carrier-molecules. The myosin-neurotubular movement is produced by ATP-Ca interaction in the same way that actin and myosin filaments are believed to produce muscle contraction. The direction of movement would depend on the orientation of the myosin molecules

vectorial enzyme reactions (possibly similar to those suggested by Kerkut 1975), axoplasm or any other substance within the axon would be moved at various rates depending on the proximity to the neurotubules.

Proof or otherwise of these theories awaits further biochemical investigation. The ultrastructural localisation of actin and myosin molecules, and a search for carrier molecules would be helpful.

Functions of Axonal Transport

The functions of axonal transport are still debated. Taylor and Weiss (1965) suggested that the amount of protein exported per day from the cyton was about one and a half times its total volume. Jakoubek (1974) produced calculations which indicated that up to two-thirds of the fast synthesis of neuronal proteins was used simply for the replacement of the natural half-life of axonal proteins. It is worth remembering that the longer axons are extraordinarily attenuated. By analogy, if the cyton of an anterior horn cell of a man's lumbo-sacral spinal cord supplying the foot muscle were the same size as that man's head, the neurone would be one mile long and have a diameter of only one-third of an inch. The volume of the axon is approximately 30 times that of the cyton, and the surface area of the axon perhaps 1,000 times that of the surface area of the cyton. The dorsal root ganglion neuron supplying a muscle spindle in a foot muscle with its central axon passing to the nucleus gracilis is twice as long as the alpha-motor neuron. Since essentially all of the protein synthetic machinery is within the cyton, it is no wonder that a very large and rapid transport of proteins and other substances is required by the cyton.

At least five possible functions of axonal transport might be suggested (see also Bradley and Williams, 1973).

1. Maintenance of neuronal proteins and axolemma.

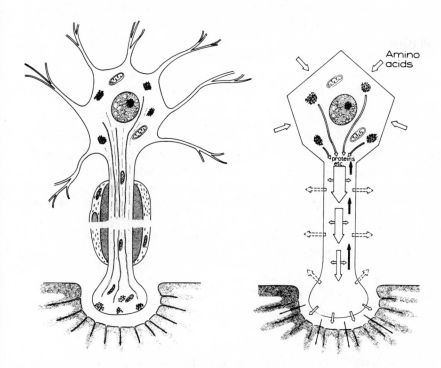

Figure 3 The features of axonal transport. On the left is a conventional diagram of a motoneurone showing the parts related to axonal transport including the Nissl substance, the neurotubules and microfilaments. On the right is shown a schematic diagram of the suggested balance sheet of axonal transport. Amino acids entering the cyton are synthesized into proteins in the Nissl substance and are exported down the axon. There they exchange with axonal and axolemmal proteins, and perhaps some pass into the Schwann cells. The amount passing in an orthograde direction thus decrements as it passes distally. Some material is released with the transmitter at the synapse, and some of this may enter the postsynaptic cell. Material returns to the cyton by retrograde transport

43

2. The transmission of information within the extremely long cell, such as that required to trigger the cyton axonal reaction following axonal section (Grafstein, 1969).
3. To provide the enzymes required for the synthesis of neurotransmitter substances at the nerve terminals such as choline acetyltransferase at cholinergic, and dopamine-β-hydroxylase at noradrenergic, neurone terminals.
4. The provision of trophic factors, which have been suggested to be responsible for such effects upon the postsynaptic cells as cannot be explained by neurotransmitter release and activity.
5. The provision of messages to the Schwan cells, such as the signal whether an axon requires to be myelinated. The evidence indicates that this signal comes from the axon (King and Thomas, 1971).

The features of axonal transport and its functions are shown diagrammatically in Figure 3. At present there is no way of measuring the value of each of these parameters. Several studies have shown that material moving by axonal transport becomes incorporated into axolemmal and synaptic membranes including synaptic vesicles (Droz, 1973; Koenig et al, 1973; Giorgi et al, 1973; Marko and Cuenod, 1973; Krygier-Brévart et al, 1974; Droz et al, 1975). The role that axonal transport plays directly in synaptic function is not certain. Blockage of axonal transport causes some of the features of postsynaptic denervation of skeletal muscle (Albuquerque et al, 1972). There are several reports of materials passing across the synaptic gap to become incorporated into the transsynaptic cell (Grafstein, 1971; Alvarez and Püschel, 1972; Korr and Appeltauer, 1974; Appeltauer and Korr, 1975; Dräger, 1975), though the amount is relatively small and its functional role uncertain.

Axonal Transport and Axonal Neuropathies

In a number of neuronal diseases, the distal parts of the axons suffer the earliest and major degeneration (the dying back neuropathies — Cavanagh, 1964). It seems likely that an impairment of axonal transport may be the basis of this distal degeneration. Most of the studies of axonal transport in axonal neuro-pathies have been performed in animals, either with toxic neuropathies causing axonal degeneration of the dying back type such as acrylamide and TOCP, or with inherited diseases of the neurone. The wobbler mouse, in which there is an autosomal recessively inherited, progressive vacuolar degeneration of the anterior horn cells, particularly of the cervical spinal cord (Duchen and Strich, 1968), has been used as a model of motor neurone disease, though perhaps its clinical course is more similar to juvenile hereditary spinal muscular atrophy (Kugelberg-Welander disease). To date the results of studies of axonal transport in axonal neuropathies are conflicting, and their significance uncertain.

Pleasure et al (1969) reported absent slow axonal transport in the dorsal roots of cats with acrylamide neuropathy, though the transport in the peripheral branches and in TOCP neuropathy were normal. Bird et al (1971) reported impairment of slow axonal transport in wobbler mice. However, Bradley and Williams (1973) found only minor changes of rate and amount of both slow and fast axonal transport in acrylamide, TOCP and vincristine neuropathies (Figure 1), and concluded that they were not sufficient to explain the neural degeneration. James and Austin (1970b) found no abnormality of axonal transport in DFP neuropathy. Bradley and Jaros (1973) found no significant abnormalities of the fast or slow transport of protein in wobbler mice. However they did find an increase in the fast, and a decrease in the slow, transport of protein in murine muscular dystrophy, where there are abnormalities of the spinal nerve roots (Bradley and Jenkinson, 1973). This finding was extended by Komiya and Austin (1974), who found a decrease in the 'super fast' (2,000 mm/day), and an increase in the fast, rates of protein transport, while Tang et al (1974) found an increased rate of the fast transport of cholesterol and phospholipids in the sciatic nerve of dystrophic mice. Jablecki and Brimijoin (1974) showed that there was a decreased rate of the transport of choline acetyltransferase in the sciatic nerves of dystrophic mice, which is transported at slow rates.

Mendell et al (1976) have recently reported a decrease in the fast rates of transport of protein in MBK neuropathy, which is associated with marked axonal swelling due to neurofibrillary accumulation. It seems likely that in all cases with axonal swellings, including neuroaxonal dystrophy, a significant abnormality of axonal transport is to be expected.

An alternative site of abnormality underlying the dying back neuropathies might be a deficient synthesis of protein and other substances in the cyton. Some deficiency of protein synthesis has been found in organic mercury p-bromophenyl-acetylurea intoxications (Cavanagh and Chen, 1971), and acrylamide neuropathy (Asbury, 1974), though no deficiency of incorporation of radioactive-labelled amino acid into the ganglia in toxic neuropathies was found by either Pleasure et al (1969) or Bradley and Williams (1973).

The Aetiology of Motor Neurone Disease and the Possible Role of Axonal Transport

Possible mechanisms of the degeneration of the lower motor neuron in motor neurone disease are shown in Figure 4. There may be some deficiency of axonal transport or of synthesis by the cyton of substances essential for the maintenance of the peripheral parts of the axon, causing a dying back type of change. There may be primary degeneration of the cyton with secondary degeneration of the peripheral axon. Less likely, though included for completeness, there may be a deficiency of the supportive function of the Schwann cell. Singer and Salpeter (1966 a and b) suggested that the Schwann cell might be responsible for the

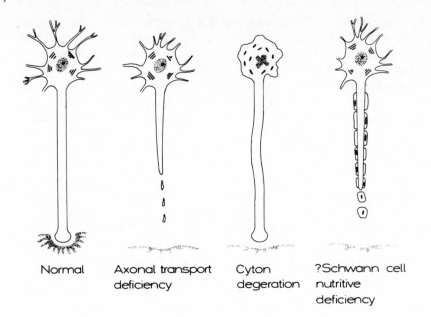

Figure 4 Diagram of the possible mechanisms of degeneration of the lower motor neurone in motor neurone disease

passage of various metabolically important substances into the axon, and deficiency of these could theoretically cause axonal degeneration. A similar mechanism to these mechanisms suggested for the lower motor neurone would underlie the upper motor neurone degeneration.

Direct study of the possible aetiological mechanisms in motor neurone disease are difficult and few have been undertaken. Genetically inherited abnormalities of anterior horn cell function are reviewed by Thomas in Chapter 5, and by Hirano et al (1967) and Amick et al (1971). The role of slow viruses in motor neurone disease are reviewed by Matthews (Chapter 12; Norris et al, 1970; Allen et al, 1971; Cremer et al, 1973). Nuclear and nucleolar changes are reviewed by Yates (Chapter 9; Mann and Yates, 1974); Kurland reviews the epidemiological evidence (Chapter 2). Other suggestions include deficiency states, eg gastrectomy and pancreatic abnormalities (Campbell, 1965; Quick and Greer, 1967; Brown and Kater, 1969; Charchaflie et al, 1974); lead and other metal intoxication (Campbell, 1965; Campbell et al, 1970; Yase, 1972); previous polio with overwork of remaining neurons (Campbell et al, 1967; Poskanzer et al, 1969; Mulder et al, 1972; Kayser-Gatchalian, 1973), as well as geographical predisposition (such as in Guam, Hirano et al, 1966) which has been suggested to be dietary in origin (Hirano and Shilbuya, 1967; Hirano et al, 1972). The relationship of motor neurone disease to paraproteinaemias and lymphomas and possibly to carcinoma has also been reported (Peters and Clatanoff, 1967, 1968; Walton et al, 1968). Abnormalities of the proteins of brain have also been described (Savolainen and Palo, 1973).

The sites within the neuron at which the underlying aetiological agent may react are depicted in Figure 5.

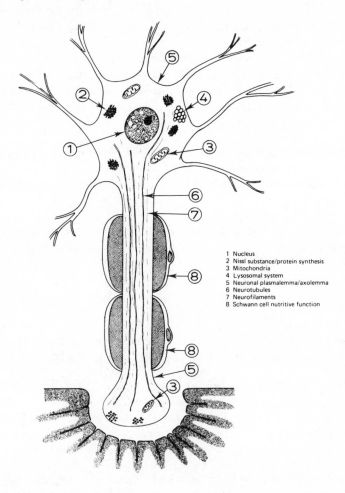

1 Nucleus
2 Nissl substance/protein synthesis
3 Mitochondria
4 Lysosomal system
5 Neuronal plasmalemma/axolemma
6 Neurotubules
7 Neurofilaments
8 Schwann cell nutritive function

Figure 5 Diagram of the possible sites of the origin of the degeneration in motor neurone disease

1. The Nucleus　Though the majority of cases of motor neurone disease are not inherited, there may be nuclear damage. A slow virus infection of the nucleus, or premature programmed degeneration of DNA, intoxication for instance with lead, deficiency states such as following gastrectomy, might all be responsible.

47

These would cause a decrease in the amount of RNA and thus of protein synthesis in the cyton, leading to deficient nutrition of the peripheral parts of the axon and possibly also a primary degeneration of the cyton.

2. Protein Synthetic Machinery   Again slow viral damage of the RNA, or the intracellular accumulation of some inhibitor of protein synthesis, toxic substances, metabolic deficiencies, or primary degeneration of the RNA might cause a deficiency of protein synthesis, with degeneration of the axon and the cyton. Alternatively if the neuronal requirement for protein and other substances was excessive, such as following polio in early life where the number of muscle fibres per surviving anterior horn cell is greatly increased, and thus the total volume of axoplasm per cyton is greatly increased, then one might expect the protein synthetic machinery to wear out before its time.

3. Mitochondria   Toxic, metabolic, deficiency or even genetic damage of the mitochondria will cause loss of the energy supply to all parts of the neurone, though the effect would be expected to fall particularly on the periphery of the axon.

4. Lysosomal System   Abnormal activation of the lysosomal enzymes by whatever means will cause endocytolysis and premature death of the neuron. This would be expected particularly to cause cyton degeneration; secondary lysosomes (lipofuscin) are particularly concentrated in the cyton in motor neurone disease.

5. Plasmalemma and other protein constituents of the neuron   Increased catabolism (or deficient synthesis) of any protein constituent of the axon is likely to cause degeneration of the whole neurone. The very high surface to volume ratio of the neurones makes the plasmalemma a likely vulnerable site.

6. Neurotubules and 7. Neurofilaments   Any abnormality of these structures or of other elements concerned in axonal transport will tend to cause a deficient supply of protein and other substances to the periphery, and a dying back type of axonal degeneration. Whether such abnormality could result from toxic, deficiency, metabolic, genetic factors or from overwork is uncertain.

8. Schwann Cell Nutritional Function   Such function is largely speculative. Though segmental demyelination is seen in the peripheral nerves of patients with motor neurone disease (Dayan et al, 1969), all the indications are that the axonal degeneration is primary and any Schwann cell abnormality incidental.

In man, studies of axoplasmic flow by measuring the accumulation of substances above ligatures in nerve biopsies or by the study of particle movements in vitro have not been undertaken in motor neurone disease. In the former case the biopsy would have to be quite long, which does not seem ethically justified. Brimijoin et al (1973) found a decreased rate of dopamine-β-hydroxylase transport in sural biopsies from one patient each with neuronal Charcot-Marie-Tooth disease, hypertrophic Charcot-Marie-Tooth disease, and Déjèrine-Sottas hypertrophic neuropathy.

Only one study has been reported of the RNA synthesis within the cyton, and that in infantile spinal muscular atrophy (Werdnig-Hoffmann disease — Hogenhuis et al, 1967). There appeared to be a decrease of RNA synthesis in chromatolytic neurons. Such studies use large amounts of extremely expensive radioactive-labelled precursors, and the number of patients required to provide sufficient data for analysis of cyton synthesis and axonal transport makes it unlikely that such a study will ever be undertaken in motor neurone disease.

A systematic study of all the possible sites and mechanisms of neural degeneration in motor neurone disease presents a major problem in man, though many are theoretically approachable. The study of all these possibilities in animal models, and the experimental application to animals of the various suggested aetiological mechanisms in motor neurone disease still seems the most fruitful field for investigation.

References

Albuquerque, E X, Warnick, J E, Tasse, J R & Sansone, F M (1972) *Experimental Neurology, 37,* 607
Allen, I V, Dermott, E, Connolly, J H & Hurwitz, L J (1971) *Brain, 94,* 715
Allen, R D (1967) *Research Programme Bulletin, 5,* 329
Alvarez, J & Püschel, M (1972) *Brain Research, 37,* 265
Amick, L D, Nelson, J W & Zellweger, H (1971) *Acta Neurologica Scandinavica, 47,* 341
Anderson, K -E, Edström, A and Hanson, M (1972) *Brain Research, 43,* 299
Appeltauer, G S L & Korr, I M (1975) *Experimental Neurology, 46,* 132
Asbury, A K (1974) *Excerpta Medica International Congress Series, No.334, Abstract No. 79*
Barondes, S H (ed.) (1967) *Neurosciences Research Programme Bulletin, 5,* 307
Biondi, R J, Levy, M J & Weiss, P A (1972) *Proceedings of the National Academy of Sciences, USA, 69,* 1732
Bird, M T, Shuttleworth, E Jr, Koestner, A & Reinglass, J (1971) *Acta Neuropathologica, 19,* 39
Bisby, M A (1975) *Experimental Neurology, 47,* 481
Bondy, S C & Madsen, C J (1971) *Journal of Neurobiology, 2,* 279
Bradley, W G & Jenkinson, M (1973) *Journal of the Neurological Sciences, 18,* 227
Bradley, W G & Jaros, E (1973) *Brain, 96,* 247
Bradley, W G, Murchison, D and Day, M J (1971) *Brain Research, 35,* 185
Bradley, W G & Williams, M H (1973) *Brain, 96,* 235
Breuer, A C, Christian, C N, Henkart, M & Nelson, P G (1975) *The Journal of Cell Biology, 65,* 562
Brimijoin, S, Capek, P & Dyck, P J (1973) *Science, 180,* 1295
Brown, J C & Kater, R M H (1969) *Neurology, 19,* 185
Bunt, A H, Lund, R D & Lund, J S (1974) *Brain Research, 73,* 215
Campbell, A M G (1965) *Riv. Pat. Nerv. Ment., 86,* 211
Campbell, A M G, Williams, E R & Pearce, J (1969) *Neurology, 19,* 1101

Campbell, A M G, Williams, E R & Barlbrop, D (1970) *Journal of Neurology, Neurosurgery & Psychiatry, 33,* 877
Cavanagh, J B (1964) *International Review of Experimental Pathology, 3,* 219
Cavanagh, J B & Chen, F C K (1971) *Acta Neuropathologica (Berlin), 19,* 216
Charchaflie, R J, Fernandez, L B, Perec, C J, Gonzalez, E & Marzi, A (1974) *Journal of Neurology, Neurosurgery & Psychiatry, 37,* 863
Cremer, N E, Oshiro, LS, Norris, F H & Lennette, E H (1973) *Archives of Neurology, 29,* 331
Crooks, R F & McClure, W O (1972) *Brain Research, 45,* 643
Dayan, A D, Graveson, G S, Illis, L S & Robinson, P K (1969) *Neurology, 19,* 242
Dräger, U C (1974) *Brain Research, 82,* 284
Dravid, A R, & Hammerschlag, R (1975) *Journal of Neurochemistry, 24,* 711
Droz, B & Leblond, C P (1963) *Journal of Comparative Neurology, 121,* 325
Droz, B (1973) *Brain Research, 62,* 383
Droz, B, Rambourg, A & Koenig, H L (1975) *Brain Research, 93,* 1
Duchen, L W & Strich, S J (1968) *Journal of Neurology, Neurosurgery & Psychiatry, 31,* 535
Edström, A (1975) *Acta Physiologica Scandinavica, 93,* 104
Edström, A & Mattsson, H (1972) *Journal of Neurochemistry, 19,* 1717
Fernandez, H L & Samson, F E (1973) *Journal of Neurobiology, 4,* 201
Fink, B R, Byers, M R & Middaugh, M E (1973) *Brain Research, 56,* 299
Fink, B R & Kennedy, R D (1972) *Anesthesiology, 36,* 13
Fink, B R, Kennedy, R D, Hendrickson, A E & Middaugh, M E (1972) *Anesthesiology, 36,* 422
Forman, D S, Grafstein, B & McEwen, B S (1972) *Brain Research, 48,* 327
Forman, D S, McEwen, B S & Grafstein, B (1971) *Brain Research, 28,* 119
Frizell, M, McLean, W G & Sjöstrand, J (1975) *Brain Research, 86,* 67
Frizell, M & Sjöstrand, J (1974) *Journal of Neurochemistry, 22,* 845
Giorgi, P P, Karlsson, J O, Sjöstrand, J, & Field, E J (1973) *Nature New Biology, 244,* 121
Grafstein, B (1969) In: *Advances in Biochemical Psychopharmacology, vol.1.* Eds: E Costa & P Greengard, Raven Press, New York, p.11
Grafstein, B (1971) *Science, 172,* 177
Grafstein, B, Forman, D S & McEwen, B S (1972) *Experimental Neurology, 34,* 158
Grafstein, B, McEwen, B S & Shelanski, M L (1970) *Nature, 227,* 289
Gross, G W (1975) In: *Advances in Neurology, Vol.12.* Ed: G.W. Kreutzberg, Raven Press, New York, p.283
Gross, G W & Beidler, L M (1975) *Journal of Neurobiology, 6,* 213
Hammerschlag, R, Dravid, A R & Chiu, A Y (1975) *Science, 188,* 273
Hendry, I A, Stach, R & Herrup, K (1974) *Brain Research, 82,* 117
Hirano, A, Malamud, N, Elizan, T S & Kurland, L T (1966) *Archives of Neurology, 15,* 35
Hirano, A, Kurland, L T & Sayre, G P (1967) *Archives of Neurology, 16,* 232
Hirano, A, Demitzer, H M & Jones, M (1972) *Journal of Neuropathology and Experimental Neurology, 31,* 113
Hirono, I & Shibuya, C (1967) *Nature, 216,* 1311
Hogenhuis, L A H, Spaulding, S W & Engel, W K (1967) *Journal of Neuropathology and Experimental Neurology, 26,* 335
Jablecki, C & Brimijoin, S (1974) *Nature, 250,* 151
Jahn, T L & Bovee, E C (1969) *Physiology Review, 49,* 793

Jakoubek, B (1974) *Brain function and macromolecular synthesis.* Pion Ltd, London

James, K A C, Bray, J J, Morgan, I G & Austin, L (1970a) *The Biochemical Journal, 117,* 767

James, K A C & Austin, L (1970b) *Brain Research, 18,* 192

Jasinski, A, Gorbman, A & Hara, T J (1966) *Science, 154,* 776

Jeffrey, P L & Austin, L (1973) *Progress in Neurobiology, 1,* 95

Karlsson, J -O & Sjöstrand, J (1969) *Brain Research, 13,* 617

Karlsson, J -O & Sjöstrand, J (1971a) *Journal of Neurochemistry, 18,* 749

Karlsson, J -O, & Sjöstrand, J (1971b) *Acta Neuropathologica, Suppl. V.,* 207

Karlsson, J -O & Sjöstrand, J (1971c) *Brain Research, 29,* 315

Kayser-Gatchalian, M C (1973) *European Neurology, 10,* 371

Kerkut, G A (1975) *Comparative Biochemistry & Physiology, 51A,* 701

Kidwai, A M & Ochs, S (1969) *Journal of Neurochemistry, 16,* 1105

King, R H M & Thomas, P K (1971) *Acta Neuropathologica, 18,* 150

Kirkpatrick, J B, Bray, J J & Palmer, S M (1972) *Brain Research, 43,* 1

Kirkpatrick, J B & Stern, L Z (1973) *Archives of Neurology, 28,* 308

Koenig, H L, Di Giamberardino, L & Bennett, G (1973) *Brain Research, 62,* 383

Komiya, Y & Austin, L (1974) *Experimental Neurology, 43,* 1

Korr, I M & Appeltauer, G S L (1974) *Experimental Neurology, 43,* 452

Kreutzberg, G W & Schubert, P (1973) In: *Central Nervous System – Studies on Metabolic Regulation and Function.* Ed: E Genazzani & H Herken, Springer Verlag, Berlin, Heidelberg, New York. p.85

Kristensson, K & Olsson, Y (1973) *Progress in Neurobiology, 1,* 85

Krygier-Brévart, V, Weiss, D G, Mehl, E, Schubert, P & Kreutzberg, G W (1974) *Brain Research, 77,* 97

Mann, D M A & Yates, P O (1974) *Journal of Neurology, Neurosurgery & Psychiatry, 37,* 1036

Marchisio, P C, Sjöstrand, J, Aglietta, M & Karlsson, J -O (1973) *Brain Research, 63,* 273

Marko, P & Cuenod, M (1973) *Brain Research, 62,* 419

McEwen, B S & Grafstein, B (1968) *Journal of Cell Biology, 38,* 494

McGregor, A M, Komiya, Y, Kidman, A D & Austin, L (1973) *Journal of Neurochemistry, 21,* 1059

Mendell, J R, Saida, K, Weiss, H S & Savage, R (1976) *Neurology, 26,* 349

Mulder, D W, Rosenbaum, R A & Layton, D D Jn (1972) *Mayo Clinic Proceedings, 47,* 756

Nakai, J (1964) In: *Primitive Motile Systems in Cell Biology.* Ed: Allen, R D & Kamiya, N, Academic Press, New York. p.377

Norris, F H Jr, McMenemey, W H & Barnard, R O (1970) *Acta Neuropathologica, 14,* 350

Ochs, S (1971) *Journal of Neurobiology, 2,* 331

Ochs, S (1974a) *Annals of the New York Academy of Sciences, 228,* 202

Ochs, S (1974b) *Federation Proceedings, 33,* 1050

Ochs, S & Hollingsworth, D (1971) *Journal of Neurochemistry, 18,* 107

Ochs, S & Jersild, R A Jr (1974) *Journal of Neurobiology, 5,* 373

Ochs, S & Ranish, N (1970) *Science, 167,* 878

Ochs, S & Smith, C (1975) *Journal of Neurobiology, 6,* 85

Ochs, S & Worth, R (1975) *Science, 187,* 1087

Peters, H A & Clatanoff, D V (1967) *American Academy of Neurology Programme, Neurology, 17,* 292

Peters, H A & Clatanoff, D V (1968) *Neurology, 18,* 101
Pleasure, D E, Mishler, K C & Engel, W K (1969) *Science, 166,* 524
Poskanzer, D C, Cantor, H M & Kaplan, G S (1969) In: *Motor Neurone Diseases,* Grune & Stratton, Inc.
Quick, D T & Greer, M (1967) *Neurology, 17,* 112
Rebhun, L I (1972) *Int. Rev. Cytol, 32,* 93
Savolainen, H & Palo, J (1973) *Brain, 96,* 537
Schmitt, F O (1968) *Neurosciences Research Programme Bulletin, 6,* 119
Schmitt, F O & Samson, F E (Ed) (1968) *Neurosciences Research Programme Bulletin, 6,* 113
Singer, M & Salpeter, M M (1966a) *Nature (London), 210,* 1225
Singer, M & Salpeter, M D (1966b) *Journal of Morphology, 120,* 281
Sjöstrand, J (1970) *Brain Research, 18,* 461
Sjöstrand, J, Frizell, M & Hasselgren, P -O (1970) *Journal of Neurochemistry, 17,* 1563
Sjöstrand, J & Karlsson, J -O (1969) *Journal of Neurochemistry, 16,* 833
Somerville, M & Bradley, W G (1976) *Submitted to Brain Research*
Stoeckel, K, Schwab, M & Thoenen, H (1975) *Brain Research, 89,* 1–14
Sunderland, S (1968) *Nerve & Nerve Injuries,* Livingstone, Edinburgh
Tang, B Y, Komiya, Y & Austin, L (1974) *Experimental Neurology, 43,* 13
Taylor, A C & Weiss, P (1965) *Proceedings of the National Academy of Sciences (Washington), 54,* 1521
Tucek, S (1975) *Brain Research, 86,* 259
Walton, J N, Tomlinson, B E & Pearce, G W (1968) *Journal of the Neurological Sciences, 6,* 135
Watson, W E (1968) *Journal of Physiology (London), 196,* 122P
Weiss, P A (1970) In: *The Neurosciences: Second Study Program.* Ed: F O Schmitt, The Rockefeller University Press, New York. p.840
Weiss, P A (1972) *Proceedings of the National Academy of Sciences, 69,* 1309
Weiss, P A & Hiscoe, H (1948) *Journal of Experimental Zoology, 107,* 315
Yase, Y (1972) *The Lancet, ii,* 292

CHAPTER FIVE

ANTERIOR HORN CELL INVOLVEMENT IN HEREDITARY NEUROPATHIES

P K Thomas

The problem of sporadic cases of progressive spinal muscular atrophy in which upper motor neurone signs fail to appear is a perennial one. The question arises as to whether they form part of the spectrum of motor neurone disease or whether they include other nosological entities. In this chapter, anterior horn cell involvement in hereditary neuropathies will be considered and its possible relevance to some cases of sporadic spinal muscular atrophy considered.

Hereditary neuropathies may be divided into those in which there is a known metabolic basis or distinctive pathology and in those in which the underlying cause is obscure (Thomas, 1975), and the latter only will be considered. These can be subdivided into three categories. In the first instance, there are pure anterior horn cell degenerations generally designated as spinal muscular atrophies but which equally well could be classified as motor neuropathies; secondly, there are instances of combined involvement of the lower motor and first sensory neurone; and finally sensory neuropathies or dorsal root ganglion cell degenerations.

The motor neuropathies (Table I) are of greatest relevance in relation to motor neurone disease and their classification has been considered by Emery (1971), Marsden (1975), Thomas (1975) and others. The most satisfactory delineation is achieved by making an initial subdivision in terms of the pattern of muscle involvement; those with a predominantly proximal distribution are genetically more complex and these can possibly be further subdivided in terms of age of onset.

The rapidly evolving autosomal recessive infantile form or Werdnig-Hoffman disease has been discussed in Chapter 1. This is a genetically distinct disorder (Pearn et al, 1973) characterised by an onset before the age of six months, often well before this time, and death before the end of the third year of life. Some uncertainty has existed as to the next category, that of hereditary chronic proximal spinal muscular atrophy. Recent studies on this question have been those of Pearn (1974) and Bundey and Lovelace (1975). The question has been as to whether the more chronic cases with a later onset can be separated into the Kugelberg-Welander form with an onset of symptoms most commonly during later childhood or adolescence and an earlier onset or 'intermediate' form.

TABLE I Classification of hereditary spinal muscular atrophies

Generalised
    Infantile (Werdnig-Hoffman)
        autosomal recessive

Proximal
    Intermediate (?)
        autosomal recessive
    Juvenile
        autosomal recessive
        autosomal dominant

Distal
        autosomal dominant
        autosomal recessive (?)

Scapuloperoneal
        autosomal dominant
        autosomal recessive (?)
        X-linked recessive (?)

Facioscapulohumeral
        autosomal dominant

Bundey and Lovelace (1975) investigated 33 cases and their families with chronic proximal spinal muscular atrophy with an onset during childhood. The index cases were subdivided into those with an onset before and after the age of two, which was tantamount to whether or not they ever walked. Most cases with an onset before two were thought to have an autosomal recessive disorder but occasional cases beginning after the age of two displayed this pattern of inheritance. From an analysis of the age of onset and disability at the age of 10 in the two groups, no evidence of genetic heterogeneity was detected. They were therefore unable to distinguish genetically between the recessive 'intermediate' form of chronic spinal muscular atrophy and the autosomal recessive disorder originally defined by Wohlfart et al (1955) and Kugelberg and Welander (1956). Among the cases with an onset after the age of two, autosomal dominant forms were encountered, and possibly some new dominant mutations were included in the earlier onset group. They concluded that approximately half of their index cases with an onset after the age of two suffered from non-genetic motor neurone disease.

The distal form of hereditary chronic spinal muscular atrophy is generally considered to be uncommon, although in a series of 200 cases of peroneal muscular atrophy and related disorders, Harding and Thomas (1976) found 21 cases in this category. The age of onset of symptoms is variable, ranging from childhood to adult life and the rate of progression is slow. The motor involvement in the legs resembles that of peroneal muscular atrophy and distal involvement in the upper limbs may become evident later. Sensory loss is not present, sensory nerve conduction is normal, as are sural nerve biopsies (McLeod and Prineas, 1971). Most cases are sporadic or show an autosomal dominant inheritance, although some may be of autosomal recessive pattern (Meadows and Marsden, 1969).

I have had a particular interest in the scapuloperoneal syndrome in which there is proximal involvement in the upper limbs and distal in the lower. Some of these cases are myopathic, but Kaeser (1965) and others have documented a form in which the underlying disorder is a spinal muscular atrophy. The onset is commonly during the second or third decades. Occasionally there is some associated facial weakness, and bulbar weakness is a rare manifestation. When the mode of inheritance can be defined, this is usually autosomal dominant in pattern, but autosomal recessive inheritance has also been suggested in one report (Emery, 1971), as has an X-linked recessive pattern (Mawatari and Katayama, 1973).

Examples of spinal muscular atrophy with a facioscapulohumeral distribution and an autosomal dominant inheritance have been reported (Fenichel et al,1967) and with a generalised distribution (Meadows et al, 1969).

Combined involvement of the lower motor and first sensory neurones, giving rise to a mixed distal motor and sensory polyneuropathy is most often encountered as peroneal muscular atrophy. As was originally demonstrated by Dyck and Lambert (1968) and subsequently confirmed by Thomas and Calne (1974), peroneal muscular atrophy can be broadly subdivided into two categories. Type I is characterised by substantially reduced conduction velocity and histologically by extensive segmental demyelination in the peripheral nerves. As this is accompanied by concentric Schwann cell proliferation around the demyelinated axons, Dyck and Lambert categorised this as the hypertrophic form of peroneal muscular atrophy. Type II is characterised by conduction velocities that are either within the normal range or only modestly reduced. As this variety probably involves a combined degeneration of anterior horn and dorsal root ganglion cells, it has been designated as the neuronal form of this disorder. Thomas and Calne (1974) firmly demonstrated that the distinction into types I and II has a genetic basis.

The clinical picture, although broadly similar in the two forms of peroneal muscular atrophy, displays a number of interesting differences apart from the nerve thickening that may be evident in a proportion of the Type I cases. This variety, for example, has a greater tendency for an associated tremor and ataxia

55

and, when ataxia is marked, such cases constitute the Roussy-Lévy syndrome. Rarer instances of the peroneal muscular atrophy syndrome include those in which there is an accompanying spastic paraplegia, others in which the motor involvement, although distal in both the lower and upper limbs, first begins in the upper limbs, and thirdly, those associated with optic atrophy. These rarer disorders are as yet poorly defined, both in clinical and genetic terms.

Patients with a combined disturbance of the lower motor and first sensory neurones occasionally show proximal motor involvement in the upper limbs and distal in the lower. This constitutes a further example of the scapuloperoneal syndrome. The sensory changes, in contradistinction to the motor involvement, display a distal distribution. The disorder has recently been designated as Davidenkow's syndrome by Schwartz and Swash (1975).

Finally, the hereditary sensory neuropathies can be subdivided into the dominantly inherited form, sometimes termed hereditary sensory radicular neuropathy (Denny-Brown, 1951), the recessively inherited congenital sensory neuropathy, and congenital sensory neuropathy with anhidrosis. The Riley-Day syndrome (familial dysautonomia) also includes a congenital sensory neuropathy as one component of its clinical manifestations. I have merely included a reference to the hereditary sensory neuropathies to make the point that these disorders are not strictly confined to the first sensory neurone as is sometimes accepted. Many cases of dominantly inherited sensory neuropathy show mild evidence of denervation distally in the lower limbs. Motor nerve conduction velocity is preserved and so there is presumably a mild accompanying anterior horn cell degeneration.

Most examples of inherited neuromuscular disorders seen by neurologists will be isolated or sporadic cases without a family history of similar disorder. This applies both to autosomal dominant and recessive conditions. In clinical practice, it is not a rare event for isolated cases of pure motor neuropathy to give rise to diagnostic difficulty, the main differential diagnosis being from motor neurone disease. Patients presenting with pure lower motor neurone involvement with a symmetrical distal involvement in all four limbs, who sooner or later also develop upper motor neurone signs and firmly declare themselves as unequivocal examples of motor neurone disease, are unfortunately familiar to all of us. Those with a protracted evolution before the appearance of upper motor neurone signs are diagnostically the most taxing, as it is not a rare event for the disorder to remain confined to the anterior horn cells for an appreciable period of time.

If the distribution of the disorder displays a distinctive pattern, such as proximal involvement in the upper limbs and distal in the lower, it is reasonably easy to be confident that the individual has one of the inherited spinal muscular atrophies. On the other hand, a symmetrical involvement in peroneal muscular atrophy, other members of the family exhibiting the more usual bilateral symmetry. Such asymmetrical cases presumably imply the operation of super-imposed environmental factors. In general, however, marked asymmetries are encountered in sporadic cases of chronic spinal muscular atrophy. A fairly typical example, is as follows:

A man presented in 1963 at the age of 30 because of weakness in his left leg which had been present for two years. For a slightly longer period he had been aware of mild weakness in his right arm. There was no family history of similar disorder and no parental consanguinity. Examination revealed slight proximal weakness in his right arm and more severe distal weakness in the left leg. His tendon reflexes were symmetrical, the plantar responses flexor and there was no sensory loss. The weakness in his left leg slowly increased and in 1968 he began to notice weakness of his left hand. At that stage he was investigated at the Royal Free Hospital. He again showed mild proximal weakness in the right arm and by this time had distal weakness and wasting in the left upper limb. The left lower leg was wasted and all muscles below the knee were severely weak. In the right leg, there was mild weakness of dorsiflexion and eversion at the ankle and of toe extension. No fasciculation was observed in the upper or lower limbs. Apart from the left ankle jerk which was absent, his tendon reflexes were symmetrical and, as before, the plantar responses were flexor and there was no sensory loss. Electromyography of denervated muscles revealed clear evidence of denervation, motor nerve conduction velocity was normal, as was conduction in sensory nerves. A muscle biopsy showed changes of denervation and a sural nerve biopsy was normal.

A diagnosis of chronic motor neuropathy or spinal muscular atrophy was made. Since then, he has slowly deteriorated, but the pattern of neurological involvement has not altered. The protracted duration of the disorder in this patient, now totalling 16 years, makes it unlikely that he will develop upper motor neurone involvement and thus fall into the category of unequivocal motor neurone disease. A recently observed case illustrates a similar clinical picture but with more rapid evolution.

A woman aged 29 presented with a four year history of muscle weakness beginning in her right hand and left arm, later involving her left leg and left arm and recently her right leg. She is now severely disabled and can only walk with difficulty. She had had no sensory symptoms and no symptoms referable to the cranial nerves. There was no relevant family history. Examination revealed generalised weakness and wasting in the limbs and some fasciculation in the left hand. Her tendon reflexes were generally depressed, the plantar responses flexor, and there was no sensory loss. Electromyography revealed evidence of denervation, as did a muscle biopsy, motor nerve conduction velocity was preserved and sensory conduction was normal.

In this instance, although unlikely, it is still conceivable that the patient will later develop upper motor neurone involvement, but a diagnosis of chronic spinal muscular atrophy is all that is justifiable. Zilkha (1962) described 10 cases from the National Hospital, Queen Square, who presented a clinical picture of chronic spinal muscular atrophy and who survived for 10 years or more. Three cases died at 10, 11 and 13 years from the onset of symptoms, and four were alive at 11—15 years after the commencement of the condition. All displayed prominent fasciculation and none had evidence of upper motor neurone involvement. He concluded that if after two years upper motor neurone signs had not appeared, a benign prognosis was likely.

The nosological status of sporadic cases of adult onset spinal muscular atrophy remains problematical. Some are likely to have a genetic basis; others, and presumably in particular those with a patchy asymmetrical involvement, are likely to be substantially non-genetic in origin. In the present state of knowledge, it is not justifiable to classify them as motor neurone disease in the absence of upper motor neurone signs. We are handicapped by the paucity of autopsy studies. It would be of considerable interest to ascertain whether there are consistent differences in the cytological features of the affected anterior horn cells as between the genetic and non-genetic cases. It would also be of value to establish whether either or both forms display changes considered to indicate an inhibition of DNA directed mRNA synthesis by Mann and Yates (1974) in motor neurone disease. As was discussed earlier, there are indications that the neuronal degeneration in the inherited sensory neuropathies may not be confined strictly to the system of neurones that is primarily affected by the disease process. This is also true of motor neurone disease. Detailed neuroanatomical assessment of cases of adult onset chronic spinal muscular atrophy may therefore conceivably demonstrate unexpected and characteristic changes in other neuronal systems.

Neurological mutants in animals, although intrinsically interesting in themselves and capable of yielding considerable information of a neurobiological nature, have to some extent been disappointing as exact models of human disease. This is perhaps not surprising in view of the complexity of the genetic permutations that are possible. Nevertheless, more detailed studies of the precise nature of the anterior horn cell degeneration seen, for instance, in the wobbler mouse, may illuminate some of the problems in human spinal muscular atrophies.

References

Bundey, S and Lovelace, R E (1975) *Brain, 98,* 455
Denny-Brown, D (1951) *Journal of Neurology, Neurosurgery and Psychiatry, 14,* 237
Dyck, P J and Lambert, E H (1968) *Archives of Neurology, 18,* 603, 619
Emery, A E H (1971) *Journal of Medical Genetics, 8,* 481
Fenichel, G M, Emery, E S and Hunt, P (1967) *Archives of Neurology, 17,* 257
Harding, A E and Thomas, P K (1976) *Unpublished observations*
Kaeser, H E (1965) *Brain, 88,* 7
Kugelberg, E and Welander, L (1956) *Archives of Neurology and Psychiatry, 75,* 500
Mann, D M A and Yates, P O (1974) *Journal of Neurology, Neurosurgery and Psychiatry, 37,* 1036
Marsden, C D (1975) In *Peripheral Neuropathy, vol. II,* Eds: P J Dyck, P K Thomas and E H Lambert. W B Saunders, Philadelphia, 771.
Mawatari, S and Katayama, K (1973) *Archives of Neurology, 28,* 55
McLeod, J G and Prineas, J W (1971) *Brain, 94,* 703
Meadows, J C and Marsden, C D (1969) *Neurology, 19,* 53
Meadows, J C, Marsden, C D and Harriman, D G F (1969) *Journal of the Neurological Sciences, 9,* 551

Pearn, J H (1974) *The Spinal Muscular Atrophies of Childhood.* Ph.D. thesis, University of London

Pearn, J H, Carter, C O and Wilson, J (1973) *Brain, 96,* 463

Schwartz, M S and Swash, M (1975) *Journal of Neurology, Neurosurgery and Psychiatry, 38,* 2063

Thomas, P K (1975) In *Recent Advances in Clinical Neurology,* Ed: W.B. Matthews, Churchill Livingstone, Edinburgh, 253

Thomas, P K and Calne, D B (1974) *Journal of Neurology, Neurosurgery and Psychiatry, 37,* 68

Thomas, P K, Calne, D B and Stewart, G (1974) *Annals of Human Genetics, 38,* 111

Wohlfart, G, Fex, J and Eliasson, S (1955) *Acta Psychiatrica et Neurologica Scandinavica, 30,* 395

Zilkha, K J (1962) *Proceedings of the Royal Society of Medicine, 55,* 1028

CHAPTER SIX

MOTOR NEURONE DISEASE:
TWO AWKWARD QUESTIONS

C A Pallis

Questions, to be fruitful, have to be put bluntly — even provocatively. While this is not necessarily the best approach in love or diplomacy it is essential, I think, in science. My questions are the following:

1. Is MND the best example we have today of what one might call 'clinico-pathological non-correlation'?

2. Do 'symptomatic' types of MND exist and,if so,do they throw any light on the pathogenesis of the 'idiopathic' form?

My answer to the first question is 'probably, yes' — to the second a qualified 'no'.

1. 'Clinico-pathological non-correlation'

In Vinken and Bruyn's (1975) monumental *Handbook of Clinical Neurology* — widely regarded as the quintessence of neurological wisdom — we find the following phrase, in the opening paragraph of the section on ALS: 'Amyotrophic lateral sclerosis is the typical specimen of a neurological systemic disease, whose semeiology is characteristic in the majority of cases and can be correlated precisely with the underlying pathological lesions'.

Such statements, in my opinion, can only be considered true if one is rather selective with the facts. Consider Figure 1. Show this to any intelligent lay person and they will be struck by the contrast between the posterior columns and everything else. Show it to a medical student or to an average neurologist and he will assume that the dark areas are abnormal and will probably say something like 'tabes dorsalis'. Now tell him that the specimen has been prepared with an ordinary myelin stain, i.e. that the posterior columns are normal and almost everything else abnormal. What is the diagnosis? The usual

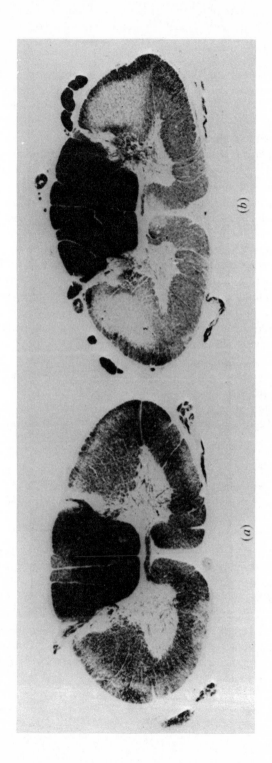

(a)

(b)

Figure 1

response one gets is 'something in the territory of the anterior spinal artery'. The figure in fact illustrates a 'typical' case of amyotrophic lateral sclerosis. It is to be found on page 639 of the latest (1976) edition of *Greenfield's Neuropathology*.

I hope this makes a point. And it should raise a number of supplementary questions. How extensive do spinal cord lesions have to be before they cause symptoms or signs? Or – more provocatively – what do we mean by a 'clinico-pathological correlation'? When it suits either our purpose or our preconceptions are we not prepared to consider far lesser changes as clinically significant? Have we thought our thoughts through when we conveniently assume that alterations of this order – say, in the spinothalamic tracts – have no clinical repercussions? Or, probing deeper still, this time into the psyche of doctors: 'what do we do, conceptually-speaking, with the sensory symptoms which, we all know, are experienced by patients with MND? Are they 'non-facts' to be swept under the carpet because they cannot readily be explained within the semantic straitjacket imposed by such terms as MND or ALS?

Ever since Charcot, many have commented about sensory symptoms in ALS. (Charcot [1886] wrote: Il est assez ordinaire que les malades éprouvent ou aient éprouvé, dans les muscles atteints, des douleurs spontanées plus ou moins vives et des fourmillements et aussi des douleurs provoquées à la pression des masses musculaires.) Friedman and Freedman (1950) said 50% of their patients experienced such symptoms. Swank and Putnam (1943) specifically mentioned pain in 'more than half' their patients. Having paid tribute to reality by mentioning these symptoms, most authorities then proceed to dismiss them as being due to cramps (even at stages of the disease when cramps are manifestly on the decline). They are said to be due to spasticity when the patient is as limp as a rag doll. Or they are attributed to a frozen shoulder joint or to thoracic outlet compression – which the patient may have, but just as often doesn't. Two things always impressed me about the great neurologists I have seen at work. The first was how they could make the patient's big toe go up or down at will. The second was their attitude to awkward or discordant sensory symptoms or signs. They would take this, omit that. This semeiology 'à la carte' may be useful when the objective is the appending of a diagnostic label. Does it help if one's purpose is real understanding?

Imagine a doctor confronted with a patient suffering from advanced MND who, in a busy follow-up clinic, starts complaining of sensory symptoms. He has to be a very good doctor indeed even to 'switch on'. He has to overcome his guilt at being healthy, and then his conditioned conviction of the 'irrelevance' of the complaints. The patient's dysarthria may preclude a probing discussion about sensory disturbances. His difficulties in standing, or in undressing, with-out aid will be positive deterrents to detailed sensory testing. Most authors describe sensory symptoms as common and signs as rare and – perhaps wisely – leave it at that.

How many clinicians, when they examine a patient with MND, are aware of the extent of the changes in the spinal cord? How many pathologists, when they look at a mounted section of spinal cord, are aware of the prominence of sensory symptoms in this disease? It is perhaps a good thing that we can sometimes get together, if only — erroneously, I think — to convince ourselves that neither matters. I can't help feeling that there is here more than a problem of communication. In the same chapter of the 'Handbook' I read that the sensory nuclei of the cranial nerves (in ALS) show chromatolysis as severe as in the motor nuclei without any apparent clinical effect. If such statements be true they constitute not only a challenge to anyone interested in MND, but to anyone interested in logical thinking.

2. 'Symptomatic MND'

My second question was of a different order. Firstly, are there 'symptomatic' or 'secondary' forms of MND? Can other conditions, in other words, mimic classic MND so closely as to cause real difficulties in differential diagnosis? And if such syndromes occur might they throw some light on the aetiology of the disease?

In real life, I don't think any of the conditions to be mentioned could for long be confused with MND. But if one examined a patient without a history — or, I suppose, a pathological specimen without a clinical synopsis — difficulties might arise. The list of conditions discussed makes no claim to comprehensiveness. It merely seeks to focus attention on some mechanisms that have, at various stages, been considered relevant.

a) *PMA following paralytic poliomyelitis* A PMA-like syndrome, coming on years after paralytic poliomyelitis, is a well-recognised entity. Zilkha (1962) reported that 8% of 133 cases of MND seen at the National Hospital, Queen Square gave a history of previous 'infantile paralysis'. With the decline in polio in the 1960s and 1970s these cases are now rare. Campbell et al (1969) stressed the frequency with which the new paralysis developed in muscles contralateral to those originally involved, but at the same segmental level. Only one of their five patients had upper motor neurone signs. The evolution of their cases — and of the cases reviewed — was rather benign. Other authors before and since (Mulder et al, 1972) have stressed these features, although most reports describe the new paralysis as being most marked in the muscles previously affected. Reports of necropsies in such cases are very rare (Steegmann 1937), in itself probably a significant fact.

I think this syndrome was too frequent and too specific to reflect the mere coincidence of two diseases in the same patient. Is there a hereditary predisposition to poliomyelitis as suggested by Addair and Snyder (1942) which might be associated with a predisposition to MND? I don't think recrudescence of the original viral infection was really very likely. I have personally seen three such cases. The CSF was always normal and the single necropsied case did not show signs of ongoing infection. The most probable explanation of this syndrome (in the majority of cases at least) is I suspect as follows. The polio virus killed varying numbers of anterior horn cells, at varying levels. The loss was not always sufficient to be clinically apparent. The patients were then abnormally vulnerable (both in their apparently 'normal' and in their paresed muscle groups) to further anterior horn fall-out, due to the ageing process or to vascular or other factors. When motor units have enlarged (through collateral sprouting) to incorporate 'orphan' muscle fibres left by their dead neighbours, the death of these particular anterior horn cells is likely to have severe repercussions on muscle power. Norris (1975) has however described cases in which such an explanation would seem unlikely.

b) *Amyotrophy following encephalitis lethargica*   Amyotrophy may occur at varying intervals following encephalitis lethargica and the literature, following the first World War, referred to a number of such cases. Their significance is that they raise the question of continuing infection.

Wimmer and Neel (1928) and later McMenemey et al (1967) reported patients with postencephalic Parkinsonism in whom amyotrophy had developed and whose spinal cords at necropsy showed not only neuronal loss but lymphocytic cuffing and neurofibrillary change. In such cases on-going infection might conceivably be incriminated. On the other hand, in the patient described by Greenfield and Matthews (1954) — in whom the parkinsonism was presumed postencephalitic (because of the association with oculogyric crises) the late amyotrophy might have been due to coincidental 'idiopathic' motor neurone disease. There were postencephalitic (neurofibrillary) changes in various parts of the nervous system but the anterior horns only showed cell loss without evidence of old or recent inflammation. What then is the relationship of encephalitis to amyotrophy in such cases? 'Propter hoc' in the first instances and just 'post hoc' in the latter? Short of another epidemic of encephalitis lethargica I don't think we can take this particular discussion further.

Acute viral infections (such as herpes zoster) may occasionally be followed by amyotrophy but the picture is unlikely to be confused with MND. Searches for elevated serum antibody titres to various viruses in patients with MND have been negative (Castalano, 1972; Cremer et al, 1973). On the other hand Russian investigators have reported progressive amyotrophy following Central European tick-borne encephalitis (Zil'ber and Soloviev, 1946; Brody, 1965).

Slow virus infection, now generally accepted as the cause of Jakob's disease, is discussed in Chapter 12.

c) *Spinal meningovascular syphilis*   This may mimic ALS (Martin, 1925). In two patients personally seen the spinal fluid was originally abnormal and the disease failed to progress following antisyphilitic treatment. One patient became a regular attender (in a subject capacity) at the MRCP examination. Both experienced sharp shooting pains in the arms which greatly assisted differential diagnosis. Endarteritic changes in the sulcal branches of the anterior spinal anastomotic chain are possibly responsible for the alterations in the anterior horn cells and lateral columns, although again little material has been available for examination by modern techniques.

d) *Hypoglycaemia* The effects of hypoglycaemia on the brain have been known for a long time, but it is only recently that experimental procedures have taken account of other contributory factors and that enquiry has included the effects of hypoglycaemia on the spinal cord. In a series of carefully conducted experiments of 'controlled hypoglycaemia' in Rhesus monkeys, in which seizures were prevented by anticonvulsants and in which acid-base status, blood pressure and blood gases were carefully monitored Myers and Kahn (1971) failed to produce anterior horn cell changes, despite the fact that blood glucose values were 'maintained below 20 mg per cent' for periods of 4–10 hours. In the neonatal rat, on the other hand, anterior horn cell change can readily be induced by hypoglycaemia (Jones and Thomas Smith, 1971). There is a problem here, concerning the relevance of these experiments to man. Patients may develop amyotrophy following prolonged hypoglycaemia, usually due to islet cell tumour (Silfverskiold, 1946; Lidz et al, 1949; Barris, 1953; Williams, 1955; Mulder et al, 1956). There has been a tendency to refer to this syndrome as 'polyneuritis hypoglycaemica' or 'insulin neuropathy' despite the fact that unequivocal anterior horn cell loss has been reported in such cases (Moersch and Kernohan, 1938; Tom and Richardson, 1951). Such patients occasionally experience sensory symptoms but sensory signs are usually absent. Recent detailed neurophysiological investigation of such a case (Harrison, 1976) confirms that damage to the anterior horn cells is the more likely explanation.

e) *Post-gastrectomy state* I have been interested for some time in the neuro-logical complications of gastrointestinal disorders. Most patients attending the medical and surgical gastroenterological clinics at Hammersmith Hospital — who have developed neurological symptoms or signs — are referred to the neurology clinic. The cases we see are many and diverse but I have not seen a single case of an ALS or PMA-like syndrome, following gastrectomy.

As pointed out elsewhere (Pallis and Lewis, 1974) the occurrence of motor neurone disease in gastrectomised patients seems to be rare. It was not reported in reviews of the sequelae of gastrectomy by Wells and MacPhee (1954), Harvey (1957) or Stammers and Williams (1963). Nor was the association recognised in a review by Stiehl (1967) of 125 patients with motor neurone disease, specially screened for evidence of previous gastric surgery. Anyone familiar with the usual practice of medical or surgical gastroenterological clinics, however, will admit that a careful search for fasciculation (or detailed testing for hyperreflexia) is seldom, if ever, part of established follow-up routine. Insidiously developing neurological disorders, especially if not associated with sensory symptoms, could conceivably go unrecognised, at least for a time. Failure to gain weight following gastrectomy is far more likely to be attributed by surgeons or gastroenterologists to malnutrition than to developing anterior horn cell disease, and in this they are undoubtedly correct.

There is a handful of reports that suggest a possibly significant association between the two conditions. Ask-Upmark (1950) described four male patients, aged between 41 and 68 years, who after partial gastrectomy and a Billroth II type of anastomosis developed a clinical syndrome resembling motor neurone disease. The interval between surgery and the onset of symptoms varied from 1 to 12 years. Because of the association of distal wasting of the upper limbs and pyramidal signs in the legs the cases were described as instances of amyotrophic lateral sclerosis. Electrophysiological data and the results (if any) of muscle biopsy (if performed) were not reported. Later, Ask-Upmark and Meurling (1955) reported three further cases and raised the question of whether a deficiency state, secondary to malabsorption, might be relevant to the aetiology of certain cases of motor neurone disease.

Kniffen and Quick (1969) published a detailed study of six patients, five of them women, who had developed various neuromuscular disorders following partial gastrectomy (this had consisted of partial gastrectomy with a Billroth II type of anastomosis in five instances, and a Billroth I type in a single case). The ages of these patients ranged from 45 to 75 years.

Neurological symptoms had appeared at intervals varying from six months to 18 years after surgery. All patients except one had visible fasciculations described as prominent in three instances. The distribution of muscle atrophy was proximal in three patients, distal in one, and combined distal and bulbar in the remaining two. Pyramidal signs were present in three patients. In two patients the reflexes were described as hypoactive and in one patient they were normal. Electromyography, performed in five of the six patients showed evidence of denervation. Muscle biopsy was also performed in five of the patients. In four it showed grouped atrophy of muscle fibres, indicating a neurogenic aetiology. In one patient there were features suggesting both myopathy and neurogenic atrophy.

Evaluation of these cases is difficult. Review of the individual protocols shows that one 51-year-old patient had absent ankle jerks, without distal motor or sensory symptoms or signs in the lower limbs. One 75-year-old woman with bilateral carotid bruits showed Parkinsonian features and evidence of mild organic dementia. Another female patient, aged 59, had well-established diabetes. One patient, not evaluated in any detail, had a serum B_{12} of only 64 pg/ml. Apart from the overtly diabetic patient, two others were considered diabetic on the basis of an intravenous glucose tolerance test and another two considered 'borderline' diabetic. Two patients showed malabsorption of vitamin B_{12} correctable by the simultaneous administration of intrinsic factor. Mild steatorrhoea, hypocarotinaemia, hypoalbuminaemia and impaired xylose excretion were encountered in various patients.

The authors considered both of the patients with bulbar signs and symptoms to have motor neurone disease and I cannot quarrel with this diagnosis. It is of interest that these are the cases with the longest latent periods (13.5 and 18 years respectively) between surgery and the onset of neurological complaints. The patient with well-established diabetes was considered to have diabetic amyotrophy. (I find this diagnosis untenable: symmetrical wasting predominated in the hands, there was no history of pain in the thighs and no comment about proximal atrophy in the lower limbs.) In two patients no precise neurological diagnosis could be made. (In my opinion these might conceivably have been instances of the proximal type of spinal muscular atrophy.)

The authors speculated as to whether postgastrectomy absorptive defects, present in varying degree in all their patients, might be the basis of the observed neurological disorders. In this context they pointed to the occurrence of pancreatic dysfunction, with consequent malabsorption in some cases of motor neurone disease (Quick and Greer, 1967; Quick, 1968). It is doubtful in my opinion whether this analogy is meaningful, as malnutrition (so often encountered in cases of chronic bulbar palsy) may itself be a cause of impaired pancreatic function (Neale et al, 1967).

Whether there is a causal relationship between malabsorption and MND, or whether their association in a given individual is purely fortuitous remains, for the moment, uncertain. It seems, however, simplistic to believe that a deficiency state, induced by gastrectomy, can be the cause of a system degeneration the progression of which is unaffected by any sort of replacement therapy. There are many neurological complications of gastroenterological disorders that we don't yet fully understand. They are not all due to vitamin B_{12} deficiency. But I don't think MND is one of them.

f) *Macroglobulinaemia*   In 1968 Peters and Clatanoff published a paper entitled 'Spinal muscular atrophy secondary to macroglobulinaemia. Reversal of symptoms with chlorambucil therapy'. A 63-year-old farmer developed widespread weakness, wasting and fasciculations, with absent tendon reflexes. There were no sensory symptoms or signs. Motor conduction velocity was normal in the ulnar nerves. There was lymphadenopathy and macroglobulinaemia was diagnosed on the serum protein and bone marrow findings. A fair neurological remission occurred after chlorambucil had been given for several weeks — with return of muscle power, disappearance of fasciculations and reappearance of the tendon reflexes. The neurological remission was maintained for a year. The underlying condition then got out of hand, with hepatosplenomegaly and petechiae. Necropsy showed some anterior horn cell fall out, 'which could not be properly evaluated due to poor fixation'. There were no changes in the long tracts. The authors postulated impaired anterior spinal circulation, secondary to increased viscosity, sufficient to cause ischaemia of anterior horn cells. The suggestion is interesting and I can personally testify to the effect of plasmaphoresis in altering the retinal vascular appearance in cases of macroglobulinaemia.

g) *Intoxication* Hypotheses implicating exogenous intoxication in the aetiology of motor neurone disease are still with us. Lead is an old contender, recently in favour again. In 1907, K Wilson had described an 'amyotrophy of chronic lead poisoning', stressing that lead could cause neurological disturbances other than acute encephalopathy in children, or acute and asymmetrical wrist-drop in painters. He described a distal symmetrical weakness and wasting with fasciculations but no sensory change. In 1970, Campbell et al resurrected this long forgotten entity. He reported that, of 74 cases of MND, 15% had a history of considerable exposure to lead. A group was identified associating such exposure with symmetrical lower motor neurone weakness and a better prognosis than in the other patients. Although blood levels for lead were normal, the urinary lead increased significantly, in the three patients studied, following the administration of EDTA (calcium disodium edetate, a chelating agent).

h) *Circulatory disturbances* It is clearly beyond the scope of this communication to review the extensive literature dealing with spinovascular insufficiency, whether in its clinical (Garcin et al, 1962; Wells, 1966; Garland et al, 1966; Henson and Parsons, 1967; Zülch and Kurth-Schumacher, 1970) or experimental (Tureen, 1936; Krogh, 1945a and b; Krogh, 1950; Gelfan and Tarlov, 1955; van Harreveld and Schadé, 1962) contexts. What might be of relevance to the present discussion however is the gradual recognition that vascular disturbances of the spinal cord — often arising from extraspinal causes, (such as severe aortic atheroma or aortic surgery) may produce clinical syndromes not unlike MND, i.e. syndromes of insidious onset and progressive course in which upper and lower motor nuerone disturbances are associated, in varying proportions, with amyotrophy, areflexia and which often exhibit a striking paucity of sensory signs (Skinhoj, 1954; Garcin et al, 1962; Jellinger and Neumayer, 1962; Hughes and Brownell, 1966; Herrick and Mills, 1971; Dodson and Landau, 1973). Such observations stress that, just as there is a selective vulnerability of cerebral structures to anoxia (well known to neuropathologists and even to clinicians), similar considerations apply to the spinal cord.

It might even be argued that vascular factors could just conceivably be involved in the differential impact of MND on cranial nerve nuclei. (The 'classically' involved nuclei have a slightly different blood supply from others — as is shown in Figure 2). I would be interested to hear of alternative interpretations for this well-known clinical observation, which may well provide a clue if not to the aetiology of MND, at least to biological differences between some cranial nerve nuclei and others.

In conclusion may I stress (Table I) certain features of MND which I think any reasonable aetiological theory will have to contend with. The disease seems to be widespread but selective disturbance of the life of motor neurones, inherited in at least some instances. But if MND is an 'abiotrophy' (see

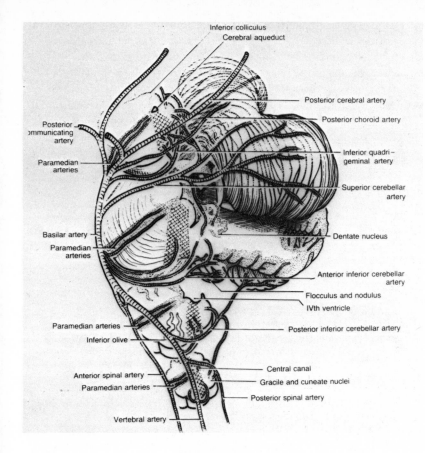

Figure 2

TABLE I Facts to be accounted for

(a) *Clinical*
 'Selective' and progressive involvement of the motor system
 Frequency of focal presentations. Asymmetry of the disease, in many cases, at
 least in its early stages.
 'Sparing' of certain motor cranial nerve nuclei, while others are severely involved.

(b) *Epidemiological*
 Very high prevalence of MND in certain areas of the world
 Positive family history in 6% of patients elsewhere
 Male preponderance in sporadic cases

(c) *Pathological*
 Occurrence of syndromes resembling PMA following spinal cord anoxia, viral
 infection, exogenous intoxication and hypoglycaemia.

69

Chapter 3) it is certainly, in its early phases at least, the most asymmetrical of all the abiotrophic disorders. To explain the local site of onset and early asymmetry of the condition I think one has to incriminate a local precipitating cause, perhaps of one of the types hinted at. As amyotrophy is not an invariable concomitant of any of the conditions mentioned, the possibility arises that these various conditions merely act as triggers, in predisposed individuals, to the development of the disease. Such a hypothesis – as perceptively hinted at by Mulder (1957) – posits the basic disorder of cell metabolism, whatever it may be, as the necessary but not always sufficient cause of the illness.

Acknowledgement

I am grateful to Edward Arnold (publishers of *Greenfields Neuropathology*) for allowing me to reproduce Figure 1 and W.B. Saunders (publishers of Bossy's *Atlas of Neuro-anatomy and Special Sense Organs*) for Figure 2.

References

Addair, J and Snyder L H (1942) *Journal of Heredity, 33,* 307
Ask-Upmark, E (1950) *Gastroenterologica (Basel), 15,* 257
Ask-Upmark, E and Meurling, S (1955) *Acta medica Scandinavica, 152,* 217
Barris, R W (1953) *Annals of Internal Medicine, 38,* 124
Brody, J A (1965) In *Slow latent and temperate virus infections*
    (Eds) D C Gajdusek, C J Gibbs, Jr and M Alpers. Washington: U.S. Printing
    Office
Campbell, A M G, Williams, E R and Barltrop, D (1970) *Journal of Neurology,
    Neurosurgery and Psychiatry, 33,* 877
Campbell, A M G, Williams, E R and Pearce, J (1969) *Neurology (Minneap.),
    19,* 1101
Castalano, Jr. L W (1972) *Neurology (Minneap.), 22,* 473
Charcot, J-M (1886) *Lecons sur les Maladies du Systeme Nerveux.* Paris:
    Delahaye and Lecrosnier
Cremer, N E, Oshiro, B, Norris, F H and Lennette, E H (1973) *Archives of
    Neurology (Chic.), 29,* 31
Dodson, W F and Landau, W M (1973) *Neurology (Minneap.) 23,* 539
Friedman, A P and Freedman, D (1950) *Journal of Nervous and Mental
    Disease, 3,* 1
Garcin, R, Godlewski, S and Rondot, P (1962) *Revue neurologique, 106,* 558
Garland, H, Greenberg, J and Harriman, D G F (1966) *Brain, 89,* 645
Gelfan, S and Tarlov, I M (1955) *Journal of neurophysiology, 18,* 170
Greenfield, J G (1976) *Greenfield's Neuropathology.* 3rd Edition.
    London: Edward Arnold
Greenfield, J G and Matthews, W B (1954) *Journal of Neurology, Neurosurgery
    and Psychiatry, 17,* 50
Harrison, M J G (1976) *Journal of Neurology, Neurosurgery and Psychiatry,
    39,* 65
Harvey, H D (1957) *Surgery, Gynaecology and Obstetrics, 105,* 559
Henson, R A and Parsons, M (1967) *Quarterly Journal of Medicine, 36,* 205

Herrick, M K and Mills, P E (1971) *Archives of neurology, 24,* 228
Hughes, J T and Brownell, B (1966) *Archives of neurology, 15,* 189
Jellinger, K and Neumayer, E (1962) *Acta neurologica et psychiatrica Belgica, 62,* 44
Jones, E L and Thomas Smith, W (1971) In *Brain Hypoxia,* Ch. 23. Eds. Brierley, J B and Meldrum, B S. London: Heinemann
Kniffen, J C and Quick, D T (1969) *Neurology (Minneap.) 19,* 312
Krogh, E (1945a) *Acta Jutlandica,* 17 suppl
Krogh, E (1945b) *Acta physiologica Scandinavica, 10,* 271
Krogh, E (1950) *Acta physiologica Scandinavica, 20,* 263
Lidz, T, Miller, J M, Padget, P and Stedem, A F A (1949) *Archives of Neurology and Psychiatry, 62,* 304
McMenemey, W H, Barnard, R O, and Jellinek, E H (1967) *Revue Roumaine de Neurologie, 4,* 3, 251
Martin, J P (1925) *Brain, 48,* ₁53
Moersch, F P and Kernohan, J W (1938) *Archives of Neurology and Psychiatry, 39,* 242
Mulder, D W (1957) *Proceedings of the Mayo Clinic, 32,* 427
Mulder D W, Bastron, J A and Lambert, E H (1956) *Neurology (Minneap.), 6,* 627
Mulder, D W, Rosenbaum, R A and Layton, D D (1972) *Proceedings of the Mayo Clinic, 47,* 756
Myers, R E and Kahn, K J (1971) In *Brain Hypoxia,* Ch. 19 and 20. Eds. Brierley, J B and Meldrum, B S. London: Heinemann
Neale, G, Antcliffe, A C, Welbourn, R B, Mollin, D L and Booth, C C (1967) *Quarterly Journal of Medicine, 36,* 469
Norris, F H (1975) In *Vinken and Bruyn's Handbook of Clinical Neurology,* vol.22. Amsterdam: North Holland Publishing Co.
Pallis, C A and Lewis, P D (1974) In *The Neurology of Gastrointestinal Disease.* London: Saunders
Peters, H A and Clatanoff, D V (1968) *Neurology (Minneap.), 18,* 101
Quick, D (1968) In: *Contemporary Neurology Symposia. Vol. II – Motor Neuron Diseases – Research on Amyotrophic Lateral Sclerosis and Related Disorders,* Ed. Norris, F H and Kurland, L T. New York: Grune and Stratton
Quick, D T and Greer, M (1967) *Neurology (Minneap.), 17,* 112
Silfverskiold, B T (1946) *Acta medica Scandinavica, 125,* 502
Skinjoj, E (1954) *Acta psychiatrica et neurologica, 29,* 139
Stammers, F A R and Williams, J A (1963) *Partial Gastrectomy: Complications and Metabolic Consequences.* London: Butterworth
Steegmann, A T (1937) *Archives of Neurology and Psychiatry, 38,* 537
Stiehl, J (1967) *Australian Annals of Medicine, 16,* 176
Swank, R L and Putnam, T J (1943) *Archives of Neurology and Psychiatry, 49,* 1
Tom, M I and Richardson, J C (1951) *Journal of Neuropathology and Experimental Neurology, 10,* 57
Tureen, L L (1936) *Archives of Neurology and Psychiatry, 35,* 789
Van Harreveld, A and Schade, J P (1962) *Journal of Neuropathology and Experimental Neurology, 21,* 410
Vinken, P J and Bruyn, G W (1975) In *Handbook of Clinical Neurology,* Vol. 22. Amsterdam: North-Holland Publishing Company.
Wells, C and McPhee, I W (1954) *British Medical Journal, 2,* 1128

Wells, C E C (1966) *Proceedings of the Royal Society of Medicine, 59*, 790
Williams, C J (1955) *British Medical Journal, 1*, 707
Wilson, S A K (1907) *Review of Neurology and Psychiatry, 5*, 441
Wimmer, A and Neel, A V (1928) *Acta psychiatrica et neurologica, 3*, 319
Zil'ber, L A and Soloviev, V D (1946) *American Review of the Soviet Medical*
    Special Suppl. 1
Zilkha, K J (1962) *Proceedings of the Royal Society of Medicine, 55*, 1028
Zülch, K J and Kurth-Schumacher, R (1970) *Vascular Surgery, 4*, 116

CHAPTER SEVEN

MORPHOLOGICAL PROBLEMS POSED BY 'MOTOR NEURONE DISEASE'

J B Cavanagh

Introduction

Three aspects of the morphology of the nervous system in motor neurone disease seem to be of importance when considering possible responsible mechanisms. These are:

1. absence of involvement of the primary sensory neurone;

2. involvement of pathways other than the upper and lower motor neurones, and

3. the reciprocal relationship between cell body and projection field in the normal situation, and in 'dying back' degenerative processes in general.

If we are to go forward in our thinking about likely causal mechanisms for this disease, these are some of the questions to which we must address ourselves from the outset. It is no longer useful in thinking that motor neurone disease is simply a disease of motor neurones, upper and lower, — it is not; the term 'amyotrophic lateral sclerosis' is less specific and more in keeping with what we know of the anatomy of this disease.

1. Absence of involvement of the primary sensory neurone

Simple inspection of myelin stained sections of spinal cord in this disease has always clearly indicated that the posterior columns are more deeply stained, and therefore contain more myelinated fibres, than the lateral and ventral columns. Even without examining spinal root ganglia, and this is not always done in post-mortem studies of this disease, it is obvious that there is no increased gliosis in the posterior columns and no loss of fibres even in the upper cervical regions, where one would expect to see the earliest changes when a 'dying back' process affects this fibre tract.

The apparent absence of change in this neurone, and its presence in many other CNS pathways, is a striking and as yet unexplained feature of sporadic amyotrophic lateral sclerosis. This cell is particularly vulnerable to attack by agents entering the ganglion from the blood stream. Unlike the CNS, spinal ganglia, in common with the autonomic ganglia, have a vascular bed which is permeable to large molecular weight substances (Jacobs et al, 1976); the sensitivity of this cell to chemicals with consequent involvement of sensory nerves in certain toxic neuropathies may be, in part, due to this easy access from the blood stream. This is almost certainly, too, a site for the entry of viruses into the nervous system and is probably one portal of entry for the poliovirus into the spinal cord.

This cell, moreover, is the largest in the body and certainly carries and supplies a larger volume of axon and terminals than any other in the nervous system. It is thus constantly involved in neuropathies where neuronal metabolism is disturbed, such as in many vitamin deficiencies and toxic situations, where we have not yet reached a full understanding of the mechanisms. Certainly the far greater volume of this cell's synthetic work seems to be a further reason for its earliest involvement in such states. It is also commonly affected in genetic disorders, e.g. Friedreich's ataxia, Werdnig-Hoffmann's disease, and it may not be too surprising to find changes in this pathway in familial forms of motor neurone disease (Engel et al, 1959). Indeed, it is this finding that makes one wonder very seriously whether some familial forms of motor neurone disease should not really be classed with the Werdnig-Hoffmann group of genetic disorders where this feature, if sought, will be regularly found (Conel, 1940).

One may reasonably ask, is the primary sensory neurone completely unaffected in this condition? It certainly shows an accumulation of lipofuscin, but this is probably not greater than normal for the age of the subject; it is always stated that anterior horn cells in amyotrophic lateral sclerosis contain more lipofuscin than normal, but there is no definitive study of this point. One also finds an occasional degenerated cell and even more rarely, a chromatolytic one in the sensory ganglia, but again, this may be no more than a normal finding, some information about age changes in human spinal ganglion cells is scanty. Wohlfart and Swank (1941) did not find any noticeable change in fibre numbers or sizes in the sensory roots that they sampled; this point should be re-examined in more detail, because their control material was one case only and taken from Swensson's (1938) study and they had no controls of their own, a serious defect in a disease affecting the older age groups. The evidence that the primary sensory neurone is completely unaffected in this disease is, therefore, not substantiated by direct studies and the clinical evidence alone is really not sufficient.

74

2. Involvement of pathways other than motor nerves

Involvement of pathways other than motor nerves has been repeatedly mentioned by many authors but never exhaustively investigated. Holmes (1910), among others, clearly showed that spinocerebellar fibres may regularly present changes and that these are more marked in the upper regions of the pathways in the medulla and in the cerebellar vermis. In myelin preparations it is not only the pyramidal pathways of the spinal cord that show fibre loss, the general lightening of staining in the other lateral and ventral regions is agreed upon by all authors. Although gliosis is most prominent in the pyramidal pathways, a little may also be found elsewhere in other tracts and seen, quite readily, if carefully sought, is the occasional occurrence of myelophages in vacuoles in the spinovestibular and other pathways indicating a steady loss of fibres. Where there is a slow steady loss of fibres in any tract, it is well known that the astroglial response tends to be substantially less than where there is a massive breakdown of fibres and this accounts for the differential gliosis picture. While the rate of fibre breakdown in these ascending pathways is less massive than in the descending pathways, it appears to be similarly of the 'dying back' type, that is it is more obviously seen in the distal regions of these pathways furthest from the cell body. It has not been generally observed, by those who have commented upon this point, that the cell bodies in Clarke's column have been conspicuously reduced in numbers. Certain features of this pathway, however, would help to explain why cell loss is not the first thing to be seen in this situation. Liu (1953) has shown in cats that if the spinocerebellar tracts are cut above the cervical bulb, the cells in Clarke's column do not degenerate but merely get smaller. This is because their fibres regularly send collaterals to the cervical bulb region before proceeding onwards to the cerebellum. This is, as Liu (1953) comments, a spino-spino-cerebellar tract, and it is not until the fibres are cut below the cervical bulb that a retrograde change with subsequent atrophy occurs in the cells of Clarke's column. The conclusion from this is that in the presence of a mild, slow, 'dying back' degeneration of this pathway, cell death would not necessarily be found, but one should be looking instead for a reduction in cell size but this has not yet been fully assessed. Similarly, in the various other tracts of the brain stem and elsewhere it is reduction in cell size, at least at an early stage, that should be sought rather than cell loss, a feature that neuropathologists do not usually seek.

A radical new approach to the topographical study of motor neurone disease may be made if we avoid the dominance of the motor pathways in our thinking, particularly since the usual post-mortem material are from cases dying two to three years after diagnosis, where the vast majority of motor neurones in the anterior horns may well have disappeared and are thus unavailable for study. I suggest that we should be looking at those pathways with a more slowly evolving change where the cells are not yet completely destroyed. This is a question of orientation and if we go on regarding this disorder as simply *motor neurone* disease, we cannot look for much progress.

3. The cell body versus the process in 'dying back' conditions

Amyotrophic lateral sclerosis has, par excellence, been an example of this type of pathological process since Gowers' description (1886). In this pathological process the largest and longest fibres are affected earliest in the disease. Clinically, this is shown in the wasting and weakness beginning in the hands and the feet in the earliest stages and progressing proximally; anatomically it is shown by the greater severity of the lesions more distally. Wohlfart and Swank (1941) also presented good evidence for selective loss of large diameter fibres in lumbar and cervical spinal roots. The same feature has been established as occurring in the cortico-spinal pathways since Gowers' (1886) first macroscopic description and there is no doubt that the longest fibres are affected more extensively in the upper neurone system. This 'dying back' process, pathologically, is one that is peculiar to the nervous system, a tissue unique in the morphology of its cellular constituents. There is a growing recognition that one of the major functions of the perikaryon is the supply of constituents for use in the very long axon and particularly in the terminals. It is becoming more generally recognised, too, that perikaryal size is a fair reflection of the size of the projection area of the cell, whether motor or sensory, and it is surprising how this simple correlation has been in the literature for so long and yet ignored by so many. Donaldson and Nagasaka (1918) clearly showed that anterior horn cells in the rat grow in size until about one hundred days of age and then stop. By contrast, spinal ganglion cells grow continuously throughout the first year of life in a linear fashion on a semi-logarithmic plot, i.e. exponentially. There is a lot of evidence in support of the dependence of cell size upon projection areas and Donaldson and Nagasaka found that there was a direct correlation between growth of body surface area and growth of spinal ganglion cell size. By contrast, it is known that while motor unit size in muscles is determined early in life, muscle fibres in the rat continue to grow in diameter until about one hundred days of age. The size of anterior horn cells, therefore, reflects their terminals rather than the motor unit or, alternatively, the number of terminals supplied by them. This relationship is well established and it is known that an increase or decrease in the size of the projection field correspondingly alters cell size. On the sensory side, Terni (1920) showed in the lizard that on cutting the tail, after subsequent regeneration, the cells of the last three surviving spinal ganglia showed hypertrophy, corresponding to their increased load of innervation, as the result of having to supply the newly grown tail. It has not yet been shown, to my knowledge, that a similar hypertrophy of anterior horn cells occurs when their terminals undergo collateral sprouting or compensatory hypertrophy as a result of partial denervation, but all the evidence suggests that such hypertrophy of the cell body will occur. Moreover, since cell size, nuclear size and nucleolar size are all interdependent, these features, too, must change with hypertrophy of the cell.

The mechanisms involved in the 'dying back' degeneration must be central to a number of different disease processes. There are, however, some disorders of the nerve cell where this process does not occur, e.g. poisoning with methyl mercury where the essential lesion is local destruction of ribosomes, polysomes and those bound to endoplasmic reticulum, in the cell body (Jacobs et al, 1975). The result of this damage is to reduce protein synthesis in the cell and so the supply of materials to the axon, effectively producing the results of axon section. Any disease, therefore, that reduces overall supplies to the axon will have this result and the effects of poliomyelitis infection are probably produced in an analogous, but more extreme, way.

The many conditions that lead to the 'dying back' process fall into two classes: those in which the cell body is directly deprived of co-factors, and those associated with the release within the axon of alkylating and other reactive groups that would tend to inactivate co-factors. The most typical of the latter group is that caused by certain organophosphorus neurotoxic substances, which have been shown by Johnson (1975 a,b) to combine in nervous tissue with a protein having esteratic properties and to release, as a result of this combination, an alkyl group. Both arsenic and thallium also produce a 'dying back' process in peripheral nerves, each probably for different metabolic reasons. Chronic thiamine deficiency (beri-beri) also produces this kind of neuropathy (Swank, 1940), while deprivation of pyridoxal phosphate from dietary causes, drug intoxication (isoniazid) or probable excessive tissue consumption of this co-factor in acute intermittent porphyria, are other conditions associated with the typical 'dying back' pattern of peripheral neuropathy (Cavanagh and Ridley, 1967). Other vitamin disorders are similarly productive of this kind of lesion, e.g. pellagra (Greenfield and Holmes, 1939).

As far as this pathological process is concerned, important new information has begun to emerge in recent years about the properties of nerve terminals that is highly relevant to this problem. Barondes (1968), amongst others, has indicated that considerable metabolic activity is taking place in the peripheral regions of nerve fibres, about which, at present, we know very little. Droz and his colleagues (1973) have shown autoradiographically that the incorporation of proteins synthesised in the cell body occurs most actively in the juxta-synaptic membranes of the nerve terminals; Heuser and Rees (1973) have shown that there is, in the motor nerve endings, during activity, a constant cycle of fusion of synaptic vesicles with the membrane and, later, reformation and recharging in the smooth endoplasmic reticulum of the terminal.

This new information begins to show us, perhaps, where may lie the metabolic activity in the distal process, towards which all the perikaryal synthetic activity is directed and perhaps, too, where the important metabolic processes, upon which the integrity of the axon and its terminals depend, are to be found. Research on amyotrophic lateral sclerosis has stagnated for too long, perhaps this book may help to show future fruitful fields of research activity.

References

Barondes, S H (1968) *Journal of Neurochemistry, 15,* 343

Cavanagh, J B and Ridley, A (1967) *Lancet, ii,* 1023

Conel, J L (1940) *Archives of Pathology (Chicago), 30,* 153

Donaldson, H H and Nagasaka, G (1918) *Journal of Comparative Neurology, 29,* 529

Droz, B, Koenig, H L and di Giamberardino, L (1973) *Brain Research, 60,* 93

Engel, W K, Kurland, L T and Klatzo, I (1959) *Brain, 82,* 203

Gowers, W R (1886) *A Manual of Diseases of the Nervous System, Vol.I.* Churchill, London. Page 329

Greenfield, J G and Holmes, J M (1939) *British Medical Journal, 1,* 815

Heuser, J E and Rees, T S (1973) *Journal of Cell Biology, 57,* 315

Holmes, G (1910) *Review of Neurology & Psychiatry, Edinburgh, 7,* 693

Jacobs, J M, MacFarlane, R and Cavanagh, J B (1976) *Journal of the Neurological Sciences, 29,* 95

Jacobs, J M, Carmichael, N and Cavanagh, J B (1975) *Neuropathology and Applied Neurobiology, 1,* 1

Johnson, M K (1975a) *Critical Reviews in Toxicology, 3,* 289

Johnson, M K (1975b) *Archives of Toxicology, 34,* 259

Liu, C (1953) *Anatomical Record, 115,* 342

Swank, R L (1940) *Journal of Experimental Medicine, 71,* 683

Swensson, A (1938) *Zeitschrift für mikroskopisch-anatomische Forschung, 43,* 491

Terni, T (1920) *Archivio italiano di anatomia e di embriologia, 17,* 507

Wohlfart, G and Swank, R L (1941) *Archives of Neurology and Psychiatry, 46,* 783

CHAPTER EIGHT

MUSCLE BIOPSY IN MOTOR NEURONE DISEASE

R C Butler, M Gawel, F Clifford Rose and J C Sloper

Introduction

In motor neurone disease the symptoms and signs reflect lesions affecting predominantly the lower motor neurone (progressive muscular atrophy — PMA),
the upper motor neurone (amyotropic lateral sclerosis — ALS) or either type
of neurone coming from the bulbar region, viz chronic bulbar palsy (CBP) if
the lower motor neurone is affected and pseudo-bulbar palsy if the upper motor
neurone is predominantly affected. In this chapter, we are reporting our findings
in 17 cases, 5 with CBP, 7 with ALS and 5 with PMA. These muscle biopsies were
studied by light- and electron-microscopy and with a variety of histochemical
techniques, quantitative methods of microscopy introduced by Engel, who with
Brooke made an authoritative analysis of muscle biopsies in motor neurone disease (MND) (Brooke & Engel, 1969), and qualitative criteria defined in a more
recent analysis of this disease by Dubowitz and Brooke (1973); we have added
a further technique, which allows the quantitative characterisation of changes
suggestive of the collateral reinnervation of denervated muscle fibres.

Brooke and Engel (1969) analysed biopsies from 99 cases, which they divided
into those with predominantly upper or predominantly lower motor neurone
lesions, a distinction not made by Dubowitz and Brooke (1973) in their analysis
of 25 cases. In both series, atrophy of Type I and Type II muscle fibres was seen
in the majority of cases, hypertrophy of Type II fibres being present in about
half the cases. A significant difference between the two series, was the occurrence of hypertrophy of Type I fibres, which was seen frequently in the first
series but not at all in the second. Muscle fibre-type grouping was seen in 7 of
the 25 patients with MND reported by Dubowitz and Brooke (1973), and in 1
of 5 patients with ALS studied by Jennekens and co-workers (1974).

It will be recalled that muscle fibres can be classified into two main types
(I and II) on the basis of their histochemical staining patterns (Engel, 1970),

these two types of fibre normally intermingling in human limb muscles to give a 'chequerboard' pattern, although changes in this pattern are seen after denervation. Cross-innervation experiments have shown that reinnervation of the denervated soleus muscle in the cat (a postural muscle consisting of Type I fibres) by the nerve to flexor digitorum longus, results in an increased speed of contraction of soleus (Buller et al, 1960), many of its muscle fibres taking on the histochemical staining pattern of Type II fibres (Romanul & van der Meulen, 1966). This work indicates that it is the frequency of impulse transmission along the motor nerve which primarily dictates the chemical properties of the muscle (Salmons & Sréter, 1976). When muscle fibres of the same histochemical type are grouped together in muscles which normally show a 'chequerboard' pattern, it is thought that there has probably been reinnervation of previously denervated muscle fibres by collaterals arising from adjacent intact nerve fibres supplying fibres of a single histochemical type.

Our findings strongly support Engel's insistence on the application of quantitative techniques to the study of muscle disease (Brooke & Engel, 1969), but this is not to decry the value of the essentially qualitative studies of Anderson et al (1967), Black et al (1974) and Achari and Anderson (1974), all of whom noted the features of denervation atrophy of muscle in MND. Quantitative techniques facilitate the recognition of denervation atrophy in skeletal muscle, especially in distinguishing these changes in slightly affected muscles from those induced by, for example, disuse or inanition. A further interesting aspect of our findings centres on the differences found in biopsies taken from patients with PMA and those with ALS.

MATERIALS AND METHODS

The patients were all seen and biopsied in the Department of Neurology of Charing Cross Hospital from 1973—1975 and those alive in 1976 were re-assessed at follow-up examination (MG). Initially there were 21 patients but four cases were excluded from the series, three because they could not be traced for follow-up and the fourth because of an atypical clinical course, namely, the disease remained localised to one limb and did not progress over a period of 7 years. The diagnosis was made on clinical grounds, the features being progressive wasting of muscles with weakness and fasciculation, with or without signs of upper motor neurone (UMN) disease or bulbar palsy. In most cases the diagnosis was substantiated by electromyography, the diagnostic pattern being reduction in spontaneous motor activity with fibrillation and large action potentials. The series was typical of others reported as shown in Table I, which compares the distribution by sex, age and clinical type.

Three clinical groups were defined on the basis of symptoms and signs as follows: patients with bulbar palsy were placed in one group, those with UMN signs such as bilaterally brisk tendon reflexes and/or upgoing plantar responses into the second, whilst the third group consisted of patients with purely lower

80

TABLE I. Comparison of Clinical Features of MND in Different Series

	Charing Cross Hospital (1976)	Mulder and Espinosa (1969)	Brain et al (1969)
No of patients	17	100	70
Sex ratio (M:F)	2.4:1	2:1	2:1
Age of onset	M 54.1 F 58.2	Mean 51.5	M 55 F 59
Bulbar palsy	29%	25%	29%
UMN (ALS)	41%	60%	–
LMN (PMA)	29%	15%	–

motor neurone signs, viz wasting of muscles with absent tendon reflexes and flexor plantar responses. As far as was possible on the clinical information supplied, the patients were grouped according to the criteria reported in the series by Brooke and Engel (1969). We also grouped all patients according to the duration of disease at the time of muscle biopsy. At follow-up assessment, patients were placed into one of two categories according to the severity of their disease; those with rapid progression to inability to work or to walk unaided, respiratory insufficiency or incapacitating bulbar symptoms, being placed in the 'severe' category. Those who had a less severe illness, and were still able to lead independent lives, were placed in a second, 'less severe' category. Because of the short duration of the disease in one woman with bulbar palsy, we were unable to place her in either category.

Open biopsies were taken from deltoid or quadriceps under local anaesthetic. Fragments of muscle were fixed in formal saline for routine microscopy in paraffin sections, and in glutaraldehyde, post-fixed in osmium tetroxide and embedded in Spurr resin, for electronmicroscopy. Cryostat sections were made from fragments immersed in isopentane and liquid nitrogen. These were treated for histochemical reactions of $NADH_2$ diaphorase, myosin ATPase at pH 9.4 (and in some cases at pH 4.6), and phosphorylase. Type I fibres stain strongly for $NADH_2$ diaphorase (Engel, 1970); they are dependent on oxidative processes for obtaining energy and are rich in mitochondria; these fibres are conspicuous in 'slow-twitch' muscle fibres, for example, the muscle fibres in the adult guinea-pig soleus (a postural muscle). Type II fibres stain strongly for myosin ATPase and phosphorylase; they are rich in glycogen and dependent upon glycolytic mechanisms for obtaining energy and are conspicuous in 'fast-twitch' muscle fibres. One hundred muscle fibres of each type were measured in their least diameter and evidence indicative of significant atrophy and/or hypertrophy was obtained by the method of Brooke and Engel (1969) for calculation of 'Atrophy and Hypertrophy Factors'.

Biopsies were further analysed with regard to the following 5 characteristics.

81

1 Target Fibres (Figure 1)

These fibres are conspicuous in denervated muscle. Experimentally they have
been seen following tenotomy as well as following denervation (Engel et al,
1966). The 'target' appearance is due to a central area devoid of histochemically
demonstrated enzyme activity (eg $NADH_2$ diaphorase), but around this area
such enzyme activity appears to be increased. Electronmicroscopy shows that this
central target area consists of disorganised myofibrils and aggregates of electron-
dense material reminiscent of Z-bands, with an absence of mitochondria.

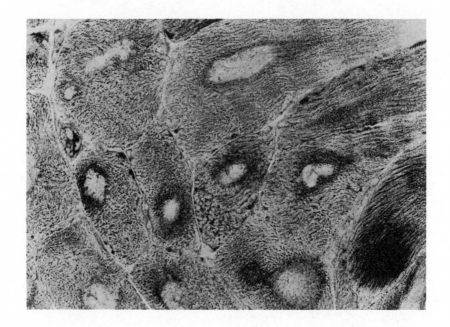

Figure 1. Target fibres ($NADH_2$ diaphorase x 400 — reduced for publication)

2 Small Group Atrophy (Figure 2)

This is the term given to the presence of small groups of atrophic muscle fibres
and is a characteristic feature of denervation.

3 Small Angular Fibres (Figure 3)

These are readily seen in the $NADH_2$ diaphorase preparation where most angular fibres give an intense staining reaction, as for Type I muscle fibres. Such
fibres are conspicuous in motor neurone disease, but are seen in other types of
denervation atrophy.

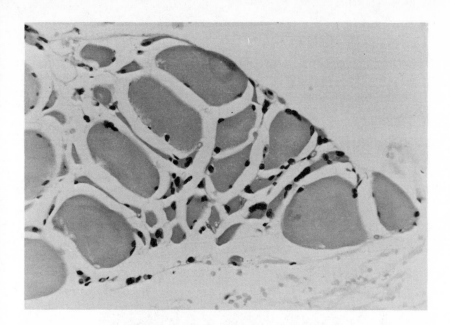

Figure 2. Small group atrophy (haematoxylin and eosin x 250 — reduced for publication)

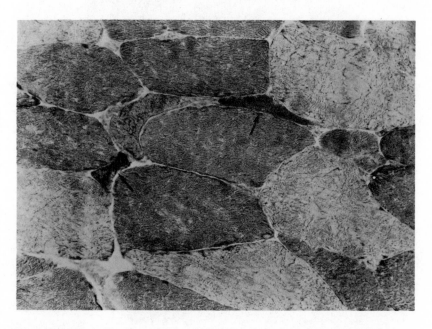

Figure 3. Small angular fibres ([arrowed] NADH$_2$ diaphorase x 250 — reduced for publication)

Muscle fibres which have lost their motor innervation undergo atrophy: some are reinnervated by axonal sprouting from nearby normal motor axons. When this occurs such axons impose on muscle fibres the enzyme characteristics seen in the muscle fibres which they normally innervate. In this way, Type I muscle fibres reinnervated by an axon supplying Type II fibres will take on the staining pattern of Type II muscle fibres. This leads to a group of Type II fibres with loss of the normal 'chequerboard' pattern of Type I and Type II fibres. The normal

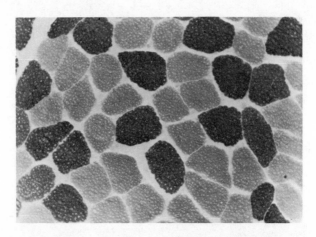

Figure 4. Normal 'chequerboard' pattern (ATPase, pH 9.4 x 224 – reduced for publication)

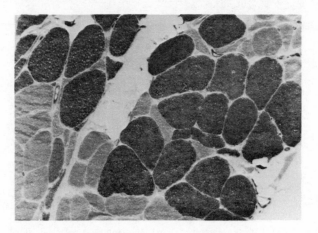

Figure 5. Grouping of Type II muscle fibres (ATPase, pH 9.4 x 224 – reduced for publication)

'chequerboard' pattern is shown in Figure 4, and fibre type grouping in Figure 5.

5 *Quantitation*

Dr Partridge of the Department of Experimental Pathology of Charing Cross Hospital has adapted from Pielou (1962) a method for quantifying the grouping of muscle fibres of a given type. In this he measures the degree of deviation from a random distribution of the two fibre types (grouping of fibre types, or loss of the 'chequerboard' pattern). Briefly, it involves recording the number of contiguous fibres of the same type (the run length) encountered along straight line transects of a transverse section of muscle. If the fibres are randomly distributed with regard to type, then the average run length of each fibre type bears a particular relationship to the proportion of each fibre type in the biopsy. Confidence limits for this relationship can be calculated from the mean run lengths and the number of runs counted. Results which lie outside these limits indicate significant departure from a random fibre-type distribution, or fibre type grouping. No comparable quantitative technique has previously been used in the analysis of muscle biopsies from patients with MND.

RESULTS AND COMMENTS

Muscle biopsies from 10 patients showed significant atrophy of both Type I and Type II muscle fibres; most showed small angular fibres, small group atrophy and target fibres, changes indicative of neurogenic atrophy. In 6 cases there was

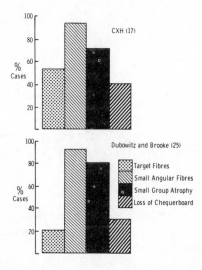

Figure 6. Comparison of morphological features of muscle biopsies. (CXH=Charing Cross Hospital)

85

atrophy of only one type of fibre, and in these cases one or other of the three qualitative features was also present; in one biopsy the presence of small angular fibres was the only abnormality. These changes are suggestive, but not diagnostic, of denervation, and similar to the series of Dubowitz and Brooke (Figure 6) although target fibres and loss of the normal 'chequerboard' pattern were seen more frequently than in their series. In terms of atrophy of Type I and II muscle fibres, our findings are similar to those of Brooke and Engel (1969), and of Dubowitz and Brooke (1973).

Hypertrophy of Type II fibres was seen in only one case but 4 showed significant hypertrophy of Type I fibres. These findings differ from those of Brooke

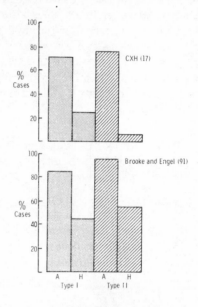

Figure 7. Comparison of incidences of significant atrophy and hypertrophy in muscle biopsies. (A = atrophy; H = hypertrophy; CXH = Charing Cross Hospital)

and Engel (Figure 7) who found hypertrophy of Type I fibres twice as often as we did, and hypertrophy of Type II fibres five times as often.

The Effect of Disease Duration

In patients whose disease had lasted 12 months or over, significant hypertrophy of Type I and Type II fibres were conspicuous, whereas this was not the case in patients whose disease had been present for less than 12 months (Figure 8). In Brooke and Engel's series this hypertrophy was clearly apparent between 7 and 12 months after the onset of the disease. Small-group atrophy and loss of the

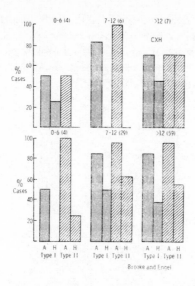

Figure 8. Comparison of incidences of significant atrophy and hypertrophy at different durations of disease (months)

normal chequerboard pattern of muscle fibre types were seen more often with increased disease duration (Table II). In the other 4 patients we could not quantitate the grouping due to the presence of many fibres which gave equivocal histochemical staining reactions with both ATPase and NADH$_2$ diaphorase.

TABLE II. Morphological Features of Muscle Biopsies at Different Durations of Disease

Months	0–6 (4)	7–12 (6)	>12 (7)
Target fibres	2	4	3
Small group atrophy	1	4	5
Loss of 'chequerboard'	1	2/3	3/6

Target fibres were seen with increasing frequency when the disease had lasted up to 18 months. Such fibres, rather surprisingly, were not found in the three biopsies from patients with disease lasting more than 18 months. Small angular fibres were present in all but one biopsy.

Biopsy Features of Different Types of Motor Neurone Disease

Most patients with predominantly upper motor neurone disease (UMN) or bulbar palsy showed significant atrophy of both muscle fibre types. Some of them

87

showed hypertrophy of muscle fibres, Type I more frequently than Type II. By contrast, patients with predominantly lower motor neurone (LMN) disease rarely showed atrophy or hypertrophy of Type I fibres; significant atrophy of Type II fibres was present in most cases whereas significant hypertrophy of Type II fibres was present in none (Figure 9).

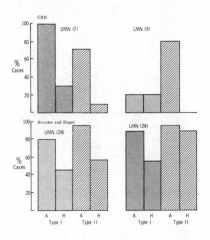

Figure 9. Significant atrophy and hypertrophy in predominantly upper (UMN) or lower motor neurone (LMN) involvement

The findings for UMN and bulbar palsy patients (Figure 10) are similar to those of Brooke and Engel but differ markedly for LMN cases since they found

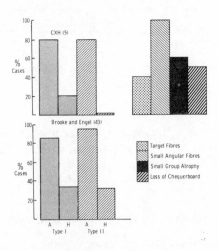

Figure 10. Comparison of biopsy features in patients with bulbar palsy

88

significant Type I atrophy, and hypertrophy of both muscle fibre types commonly.
There were other morphological differences between UMN and LMN cases (Figure
11), viz small group atrophy was seen much more frequently in the cases with
upper motor neurone involvement than in those with *lower* motor neurone involvement. Loss of the chequerboard pattern — possibly evidence of collateral

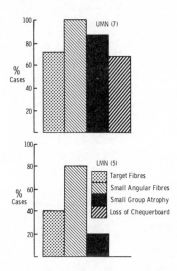

Figure 11. Morphological features of biopsies from patients with predominantly upper or
lower motor neurone involvement

re-innervation — was also seen more frequently in the patients with UMN disease.
The patients with bulbar palsy were intermediate with regard to these features.

Severity of Muscle Weakness

With a view to discovering the earliest histological manifestation of MND, biopsies were taken in four patients from two different muscles on the same day, one
muscle being severely affected, the other less so. The muscles differed in that
target fibres were seen in 3 of 4 severely affected muscles, but none was seen in
the less affected muscles (Table III).

Severity of Disease

At the time of follow-up assessment, patients were placed into one of two categories according to the severity of their disease, as described below.

Muscle fibre hypertrophy was seen in 5 of 9 patients with the milder form of
the disease, but in none of those with the severe form of the disease. Moreover,

89

TABLE III. Comparison of Biopsies Taken from Severely and Less Severely Affected Muscles at Same Time

	Severely affected (4)	Less severely affected (4)
Type I fibres		
Atrophy	4	4
Hypertrophy	1	2
Type II fibres		
Atrophy	4	4
Hypertrophy	0	1
Target fibres	4	0
Small angular fibres	4	4
Small group atrophy	3	2
Loss of chequerboard	1	1

4 of 7 of the former compared with only one of 5 of those with severe disease showed a loss of the chequerboard pattern, that is, evidence suggestive of collateral re-innervation. (Figure 12).

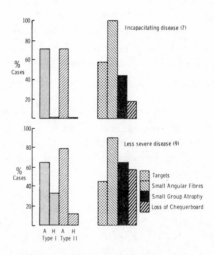

Figure 12. Comparison of biopsies taken from patients with severe and less severe disease course

DISCUSSION

Recent investigations of muscle biopsies in *motor neurone disease* have involved the application of new cytochemical techniques and quantitative histological procedures, largely pioneered by Engel. These procedures have not only modified the criteria by which denervation atrophy has been characterised in earlier studies of motor neurone disease (see for example Anderson et al, 1967), but have revealed a number of other interesting and as yet unexplained features, the most important being the presence of hypertrophied muscle fibres, which are presumably compensating for the neurogenic atrophy of muscle typically found in the disease. Instead of the chequerboard pattern of Type I and Type II muscle fibres normally found in human muscle, there is a tendency for muscle fibres of a given type to be grouped together. This change probably reflects the collateral re-innervation of atrophic fibres by nerve-buds arising from adjacent and unaffected nerve fibres supplying muscle of a single fibre type.

With regard to the methods used in these investigations, our own correspond closely to those introduced by Brooke and Engel (1969) particularly with regard to the characterisation of abnormal degrees of atrophy or hypertrophy of muscle fibres. As these workers showed so conclusively, it is the range of fibre-size and not the mean muscle fibre-diameter which is important. They concentrated on such measurements in 99 cases of motor neurone disease categorising what can loosely be termed 'fast' and 'slow' fibres in terms of 'strong' (Type II) and 'weak' (Type I) reactions with myosin ATPase. Dubowitz and Brooke's (1973) measurements are based on the same techniques, save that the myosin ATPase reaction was performed at pH 4.6 as well as at 9.4, to distinguish II.A and II.B fibres. This step we have taken in a few cases; and we have also performed our measurements on sections stained not only with myosin ATPase (pH 9.4), but also with $NADH_2$ diaphorase, an oxidative enzyme present in high concentration in Type I fibres. We have not yet fully assessed the advantages implicit in using these two techniques for our measurements. To identify a fibre as Type I in that it does *not* react strongly with myosin ATPase at pH 9.4 is somewhat unsatisfactory, and especially so when muscle fibres are atrophic or otherwise abnormal. It should be added that in most of our 17 cases we have also distinguished Type II fibres by what is probably the most cytochemically meaningful technique for this purpose, namely by demonstrating their high content of phosphorylase.

We have introduced, too, a method which allows us to quantitate the extent to which the normal chequerboard pattern of Type I and Type II fibres is replaced by a pattern in which muscle fibres of a single type are arranged in groups, which thus suggests collateral re-innervation. This is likely to have wide applications.

With regard to qualitative changes indicative of denervation atrophy, we have paid close attention to those features stressed by Dubowitz and Brooke (1973) in their analysis of 25 biopsies from motor neurone disease.

In our series strong evidence of denervation atrophy — small group atrophy and atrophy of both muscle fibre types — was present in 12 of 17 cases, and less conclusive evidence in the remaining 5. This proportion is similar to that reported by Brooke and Engel (1969) and Dubowitz and Brooke (1973). Like these workers we found no changes which would distinguish the muscle atrophy seen in motor neurone disease from that encountered in other forms of neurogenic atrophy. We had incidentally hoped that a comparison between biopsies taken from less and more affected muscles in 4 individual patients might enable us to recognise early and perhaps specific features of MND, but this did not prove to be the case.

Significant hypertrophy of muscle fibres was also present, but there are curious differences between our findings and those of Brooke and Engel, and between those of Brooke and Engel and those of Dubowitz and Brooke. Thus Brooke and Engel and Dubowitz and Brooke reported significant hypertrophy of Type II fibres in just over half of the cases analysed, a change we found in only one of our cases. Yet in terms of duration of disease and age and sex incidence, and again in terms of the proportion of cases with predominantly upper motor neurone (ALS) or lower motor neurone (PMA) involvement, our series corresponds with that of Brooke and Engel. (The relevant clinical information with regard to ALS and PMA is not given in Dubowitz and Brooke's analysis.) With regard to hypertrophy of Type I fibres, Brooke and Engel reported this in half their cases, Dubowitz and Brooke in none of theirs, whilst we found it to be present in a quarter of our cases. Dubowitz and Brooke commented on the discrepancy between their findings and those of Brooke and Engel, tentatively attributing this to the shorter duration of disease in their cases (less than 12 months). Our findings do not support this explanation since 2 of our 12 patients with a disease duration of less than 12 months showed Type I fibre hypertrophy.

There was a suggestion in our series that compensatory hypertrophy of muscle fibres might be of prognostic significance in MND. Such hypertrophy was present in 5 of 9 patients who had the less severe form of the disease, but was not seen in any of the 7 patients who had severe disease. This hypertrophy was of Type I fibres in 4 cases and Type II in one. Whatever the case, we propose to see whether the patterns of muscle fibre hypertrophy seen in MND may be of value in distinguishing this condition from other forms of neurogenic muscle atrophy.

With regard to muscle fibre-type grouping, this has usually been assessed subjectively. With our quantitative method we found significant grouping in 6 of 13 cases of MND. This is a higher proportion than that (7 in 25) observed by Dubowitz and Brooke, or again, by Jennekens et al (1974) who noted fibre type grouping (more than 15 Type I or Type II fibres together) in 1 of 5 cases of ALS. Such grouping was present in 4 of the 7 patients who had the less severe form of the disease, but in only 1 of the 5 patients with the severe form. This suggests that the presence of collateral re-innervation may also be of prognostic significance in MND. Fibre-type grouping was noted in 4 of 5 cases of ALS and in 2 of 4 cases of chronic bulbar palsy, but was lacking in 4 cases of PMA. It is possible, therefore, that there is a failure of collateral re-innervation in PMA, a point which merits further investigation in a larger series of cases.

Summary

In 17 patients with motor neurone disease, biopsies from proximal muscle of either upper or lower limb have been examined.

Patterns of muscle fibre change were studied by histological and quantitative histochemical techniques. These included a new method for the identification of significant grouping of Type I or Type II fibres, a change which probably represents re-innervation of denervated muscle fibres.

A pattern of muscle fibre atrophy indicative of denervation atrophy was seen in 12 cases, a proportion similar to that seen in other series. Evidence of denervation was less definite in the remaining cases.

Evidence of collateral re-innervation was found in the majority of cases with amyotrophic lateral sclerosis (ALS) but in no cases of progressive muscular atrophy (PMA). This unexpected finding, if confirmed in a large series of patients, may imply a difference in the motor neurone lesion encountered in ALS and PMA.

Significant muscle fibre hypertrophy, probably a compensatory phenomenon, was found in 5 cases. Such hypertrophy and evidence of collateral re-innervation appear to be correlated with a better prognosis.

References

Achari, AN and Anderson, MS (1974) *Neurology, 24,* 477

Anderson, PJ, Song, SK, Slotwiner, P (1967) *Journal of the Mount Sinai Hospital, 34,* 171

Black, JT, Bhatt, GP, Dejesus, PV, Schotland, DL and Rowland, LP (1974) *Journal of Neurological Sciences, 21,* 59

Brain, WR, Croft, PB and Wilkinson, M (1969) In *Motor Neurone Diseases.* (Ed) LH Norris and LT Kurland. Grune and Stratton, New York. Page 20

Brooke, MH and Engel, WK (1969) *Neurology, 19,* 221 and 378

Buller, AJ, Eccles, JC and Eccles, RM (1960) *Journal of Physiology, 150,* 417

Dubowitz, V and Brooke, MH (1973) *Muscle Biopsy: A Modern Approach.* WB Saunders, London. Page 107

Engel, WK (1970) *Archives of Neurology, 22,* 97

Engel, WK, Brooke, MH and Nelson, PG (1966) *Annals of the New York Academy of Science, 138,* 160

Jennekens, FGI, Meijer, AEFH, Bethlem, J and van Wijngaarden, GK (1974) *Journal of Neurological Sciences, 23,* 337

Mulder, DW and Espinosa, RE (1969) In *Motor Neurone Diseases.* (Ed) (Ed) LH Norris and LT Kurland. Grune and Stratton, New York. Page 12

Pielou, EC (1962) *Biometrics, 18,* 579

Romanul, FCA and van der Meulen, JP (1966) *Nature, 212,* 1369

Salmons, S and Sréter, FA (1976) *Nature, 263,* 30

CHAPTER NINE

NEURONAL CHANGES IN MOTOR NEURONE DISEASE

P O Yates

Qualitative description of morphological change is the essence of pathology even today. Opinions and hypotheses are offered from an intuitive feeling that the observed objects are darker or smaller or more numerous than the pathologist's previous experience — a state of affairs entirely familiar to the daily practice of clinicians. Measuring and counting things does not improve vision greatly but it concentrates observation remarkably and allows opinions to be given (or refuted) with greater confidence. What then are the qualitative changes that we see in the nervous system in motor neurone disease?

Pathologically, there is a loss of motor cells from anterior horns of the spinal cord, motor nuclei of brainstem and motor cortex, and degenerative changes in remaining cells of these areas. In affected but surviving cells the cell body is usually shrunken and may appear to contain excessive amounts of lipofuscin. This is probably because the Nissl granules (RNA) are often lost and what remains is conglomerated into masses which lie near the cell membrane. Nuclear changes are common; the chromatin, which is relatively inconspicuous in normal cells, is prominent and, in severely diseased neurones, the nucleus is usually shrunken and heterochromatic, while even in mildly affected cells some chromatin clumping is seen.

We have attempted a quantitative study of these changes in motor neurones in the hope that the earliest stage of the disease process could be identified. Observations were made on a case of motor neurone disease (case A) which was of only four months' duration and was prematurely terminated as a result of accidental death, and compared with those made on a long-standing case of motor neurone disease (case B) and a normal control free from neurological illness (case C). In the first case it was thought possible that the disease had not progressed to such an extent that all affected cells would be in an advanced atrophic condition, and early pathological changes might still be present in some cells.

A brief summary of the clinical history and neuropathology of both MND cases now follows.

CASE A

Clinical History At the age of 77 years the patient developed a weakness of the left arm and hand which rapidly spread to involve the right arm and both legs. He was found to have wasting and weakness of the muscles of the left arm, and widespread fasciculation of all muscles of the arms and legs. Power was markedly diminished in the left arm and shoulder and slightly less so in the right arm and flexors of the hips and knees. There was wasting of the small muscles of both hands (left greater than right), and the patient had difficulty in using the fingers. Right facial weakness was seen, but otherwise the cranial nerves showed no abnormality.

Two months later the limb muscles had so weakened that the patient had severe difficulty in walking. Fasciculation of the tongue was present, but no further cranial nerve involvement was seen. Electromyographic studies were consistent with a diagnosis of motor neurone disease. Shortly afterwards the patient was admitted to hospital after a road accident. He did not respond to treatment and died of bronchopneumonia without regaining consciousness.

CASE B

The patient was first examined at the age of 42 years with an 18 month history of tremor of the left arm and leg. Since then she had developed a tendency to drag her right foot. By two years before her death she had severe limb weakness of arms and legs. She was found to have bilateral facial weakness and bulbar palsy, which caused much difficulty in speaking and swallowing. There was gross wasting of the neck muscles, such that she was unable to extend her head. There was marked weakness, wasting and fasciculation of all limb muscles, especially in the arms. No abnormality of sensation was noted. Electromyographic studies revealed widespread denervation in all limbs. She was admitted to hospital with severe difficulty in eating, speaking and coughing; she continued to deteriorate until her death at the age of 52 years.

Pathological findings In both cases all findings in muscles and nervous system were consistent with the diagnosis of motor neurone disease. The most severe changes were seen in the anterior horn cells of the spinal cord (especially the ventromedial cell column), Betz cells of cerebral cortex and cells of the hypo-glossal nucleus. Remaining cells in these areas were in an advanced state of degeneration; many of them were completely shrunken, showing a great loss of Nissl substance. The nucleus was severely shrunken and in many cells the chromatin was represented by a few large heterochromatic granules. The nucleolus was either absent or severely atrophied.

The motor neurones of the cranial nerve nuclei were better preserved but all showed abnormalities; changes in the cells of the VI, VII, VIII and XII nuclei being more severe than in the III, IV and V nuclei. In the oculomotor and trigeminal nerve nuclei of both cases cells of normal appearance were seen scattered among obviously diseased neurones. This was especially so in Case A (the case dying accidentally). Diseased neurones showed a variety of changes. In early stages the nucleus was sometimes slightly shrunken, in which case the chromatin was often clumped into heterochromatic granules; the nucleolus was, however, normally stained. Nissl granules were either unaltered or fine and powdery centrally, while larger granules were peripherally sited.

More severely damaged cells showed loss of Nissl granules, the remainder being clumped into large masses. The nucleolus showed altered staining and the nuclear chromatin was shrunken. Later still the nuclear DNA was represented by a few heterochromatic clumps and the nucleolus was either degenerate or absent. Finally, the remaining cytoplasm had lost all nucleic acids and contained only the hydrolytically resistant lipofuscin granules.

Such a mixed population containing normal and diseased cells was, therefore, ideal for the following quantitative study.

METHODS

Nervous tissue was obtained at necropsy from both MND and control cases within 12 hours of death. The results of an autolysis experiment showed that during a period of 11 hours of refrigerated storage after death, nervous tissue lost the majority of low molecular weight RNA species (transfer, nuclear and messenger RNA which could not therefore be studied) but no cytoplasmic or ribosomal RNA (Nissl substance) which constitutes about 70% of the total nor any DNA.

We calculated nuclear volumes and nucleolar volumes, measured amounts of nuclear DNA and cytoplasmic RNA in neurones from a wide variety of sites in cord, brain-stem and cerebral cortex.

It will be best to indicate at this point our reasoning that led us to make these observations. We were concerned to look at the structural features that might be indicators of a cell's capacity for metabolic activity. Obviously in examining post mortem human tissue we could derive no information about the rate of metabolism or indeed the presence or absence of cell function in life.

DNA seems to be present in the same quantities in all mature cells of a species even though it appears that only 5–10% is referred to in adult tissue. Redundant DNA may have been concerned with cell differentiation and early maturation. However, the size of cell nuclei varies greatly from tissue to tissue as does the openness and apparent dispersal of the chromosome material. Nuclear size seems to be related to total protein output of the cell both for its own maintenance and for external secretion. Perhaps the open nucleoplasm is better able to form and pass the large quantities both of messenger RNA which instruct the ribosomes of the cytoplasm as to protein creation and of the large amounts of the simpler transfer RNA that locate and carry the required aminoacids.

The nucleolus is the principal site of creation of RNA for the ribosomes which, passing into the cytoplasm, becomes the Nissl substance on which proteins are formed.

There is, therefore, a nucleolar/ribosomal RNA aspect of a cell which represents a general capacity to form protein and a separate nuclear activity providing the information as to which protein should be formed. Motor neurones normally have very large nuclei and nucleoli and an amount of cytoplasmic RNA appropriate to the largest cells in the body.

Firstly we did not find any change in the quantity of DNA in the nuclei of the motor neurone disease cases until final cell disintegration had begun. There was a redistribution of the chromosomal material which formed large clumps close to the nuclear membrane. The earliest change in any of our measurements was a reduction in nuclear volume with some irregularities of outline.

There are variations between the nerve cells of a particular group in nuclear size but normally a very close correlation between several of the factors was measured. This correlation to some extent characterises a group of neurones and doubtless mirrors their very similar metabolism and function. If, for example,

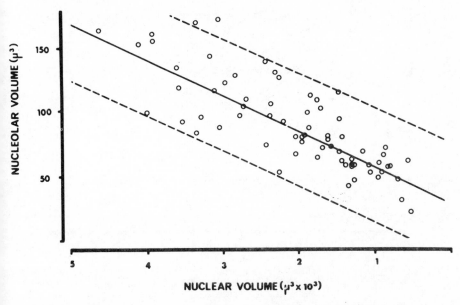

Figure 1   Correlation of nuclear and nucleolar volumes for motor cells of the anterior horns in the control case

97

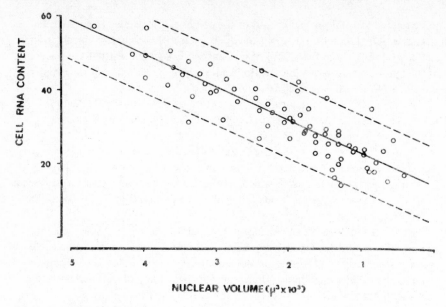

Figure 2   Relationship of nuclear volume and cytoplasmic (ribosomal) RNA for anterior horn cells of control case

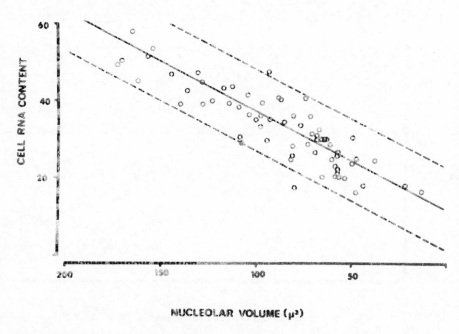

Figure 3   Relationship of nucleolar volume and cytoplasmic (ribosomal) RNA for anterior horn cells of control case

we look at normal anterior horn cells at one spinal cord level there is quite a good relationship between the size of a nucleus and of its nucleolus and between each of these factors and the quantity of cytoplasmic RNA or Nissl substance (Figures 1, 2, 3).

Both the MND cases show differences from these normal patterns. It was notable that in the long-standing MND case (B) the proportion of cells showing shrunken nuclei in a less severely affected nerve group such as the trigeminal motor nucleus is greater than that in the accidentally terminated case A, whereas in severely affected cell groups such as anterior horn cells both cases show that all cells contain shrunken nuclei. This variation in degree of the disease process allowed us a cross sectional view of what we believe is the time sequence of change.

Nucleolar volume and ribosomal RNA maintained the normal close linear relationship even in moderately diseased cell groups of Case A such as the motor neurones of the trigeminal where the cells had begun to show nuclear shrinkage.

Plotting nuclear volume against ribosomal RNA for the same group of cells shows this feature (Figure 4). The reduction of nuclear volume proceeds to a level of about 1000 cu μ is attained when cell disintegration begins.

Nucleolar volume and cytoplasmic RNA remain normal whilst the early stages

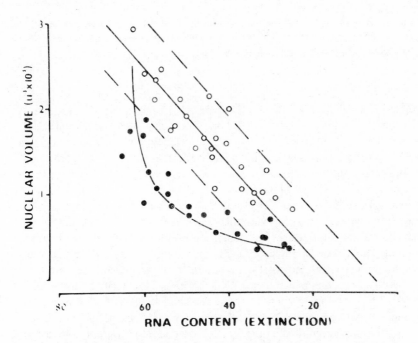

Figure 4 Graph of relationship of cytoplasmic (ribosomal) RNA and nuclear volume for trigeminal motor cells of case A. Filled circles represent cells with nuclear disease changes

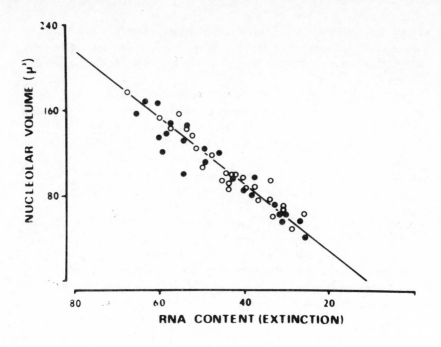

Figure 5   Graph showing the persistant relationship between nucleolar volume and cytoplasmic (ribosomal) RNA even for cells with shrunken nuclei (filled circles). Motor cells of trigeminal nucleus, case A

of nuclear shrinkage takes place. After a certain level of nuclear change the nucleoli also begin to get smaller and the cytoplasmic RNA also diminishes proportional to nucleolar reduction until a nucleolar minimal volume is reached whereafter the RNA disappears completely as cell death occurs (Figure 5).

Our interpretation of these changes is that the initial site of action of the MND pathogen is the nucleus and its prime effect is to cause (either directly or indirectly) a decrease in nuclear volume accompanied by a condensation of the chromatin nucleoprotein, but without a concomitant loss of DNA and, furthermore, initially without effect on nucleolar appearance or the cytoplasmic RNA content. The DNA is presumably inactivated, being changed structurally from a metabolically available diffuse form into a relatively inactive dense form with a consequent reduction in messenger RNA synthesis (Hsu, 1962; Littau et al, 1964). This reduction in nuclear volume and condensation of DNA proceeds with little effect on the cell's metabolic capacity, as indicated by a normally active nucleolus and normal cytoplasmic ribosomal RNA content, until a volume of 1000 μm^3 is reached. At this point, the nucleolus also shrinks and cytoplasmic RNA begins to disappear from the cell, (Mann & Yates, 1974).

100

Since cell protein synthesis is dependant upon the rapid turnover of a small pool of messenger and transfer RNA molecules (Koenig, 1968) derived from the nucleus, once supplies of these are reduced, cell synthetic activity will soon diminish. This will result in a failure to supply the cell with the essential protein (enzymes, membrane glycoprotein, tubulin, etc.) necessary to maintain its metabolic economy.

References

Hsu, H (1962) *Experimental Cell Research, 7,* 332
Koenig, H (1968) In *Motor Neurone Diseases*, Ed. F.H. Norris Jr and
    L T Kurland, Grune and Stratton: New York, p. 347
Littau, V C, Allfrey, V C, Frenster, J H and Mirsky, A E (1964) *Proceedings of the National Academy of Sciences of the United States of America, 52,* 93
Mann, D M A and Yates, P O (1974) *Journal of Neurology, Neurosurgery, and Psychiatry, 37,* 1036

CHAPTER TEN

NEUROFIBRILLARY CHANGES IN A PARTICULAR TYPE OF MOTOR NEURONE DISEASE

J Trevor Hughes

It is now evident from many published reports that some human neuronal disorders are accompanied by certain distinctive neurofibrillar changes seen both in the perikarya and in the axons and found, not only in the neurones of the central nervous system, but also in the peripheral neurones of the sensory and autonomic ganglia. The research work on which these findings have been based has been made possible by the development of electron-microscopical techniques allowing the ultrastructural study of individual neurones, first in experimental conditions and then in human diseases. A notable landmark was the work of Kidd (1963) and Terry (1963) who demonstrated with the electron microscope that the neurofibrillary tangle of Alzheimer's disease was made up of abnormal neurofilaments. Similar abnormal filaments to those seen in Alzheimer's disease have subsequently been found in the inherited neurological disease prevalent on Guam Island (Hirano et al, 1966), Pick's disease (Schochet et al, 1968) and post-encephalitic Parkinsonism (Wisniewski et al, 1970). This list of diseases with neurofibrillary pathology is not exhaustive and, at the 1976 meeting of the American Association of Neuropathologists, papers were ready which described abnormal neurofibrillary pathology in cases of subacute sclerosing panencephalitis and in cases of cerebral vascular malformations, where neurofibrillary changes were found adjacent to angiomata.

The interest in the ultrastructural changes found in these diseases has extended the search for similar changes in various experimental conditions. Thus the intracerebral injection of alum phosphate (Klatzo et al, 1965) was found to produce striking neuronal changes throughout the central nervous system. The alkaloids colchicine, podophyllotoxin, vinblastine, and vincristine, all of which belong to the class of metaphase-blocking antimitotic drugs, have also been found to cause neurofibrillary degeneration in experimental animals and in human patients undergoing treatment for malignant disease (Wisniewski et al, 1968). Other experimental degenerations such as lathyrogenic encephalopathy, vitamin E deficiency, and copper deficiency have produced similar changes (Wisniewski et al, 1970).

The finding of neurofibrillary change in motor neurone disease was first reported by Carpenter (1968). Carpenter used the electron microscope to investigate axonal enlargements which he found in cases of sporadic motor neurone disease. Although his observations were mainly directed to the nature of the axonal swellings he did describe similar material within the perikarya of the motor neurones. Electron microscopy of the enlarged axons showed them to be distended by neurofilaments, which were not described in detail and no measurement of the filaments were given. Schochet et al (1969) described similar intracytoplasmic material distending the motor neurones of the spinal cord and of the brain stem in a case of sporadic motor neurone disease. The ultrastructural examination of the abnormal material showed it to consist of bundles of parallel neurofilaments whose diameter was estimated at 10 nm. These two papers stimulated a search for neurofibrillary changes in the neurones of cases of motor neurone disease and also in variants of this condition.

Amongst atypical forms of motor neurone disease are cases in which an inherited neurological disorder originally classified as familial amyotrophic lateral sclerosis differs in certain important details from both the familial and sporadic forms of motor neurone disease. This particular condition was referred to by Kurland and Mulder (1955) and by Engel et al (1959) but a full pathological description was given by Hirano et al (1967). All the pathological features of motor neurone disease are present including cortico-spinal tract degeneration, depletion or absence of the spinal motor neurones, atrophy of the anterior spinal nerve roots, and denervation changes in the skeletal muscles. In addition to this group of findings, which are characteristic of motor neurone disease, the cases have degeneration of the posterior white columns and of both the anterior and posterior spino-cerebellar tracts. Clarke's column (nucleus dorsalis) is severely degenerated. One of the very interesting features of this condition was the presence in many of the surviving anterior horn motor neurones of hyaline intracytoplasmic inclusion material. There has been considerable interest in the nature of this intracytoplasmic material whose ultrastructure had not been examined. A further case of this disease with observations on the ultrastructure was made by Hughes and Jerrome (1970) and the following account is based on their report.

CASE REPORT

Clinical History

A woman aged 64 years had, for the twenty years before her death, suffered from weakness of both legs with bilateral foot drop. She also had weakness of the small muscles of the hands and an unsteady gait suggestive of ataxia. Sensation was otherwise normal. Fasciculation was present in both upper and lower limb muscles. Electromyography showed the pattern of changes found in motor neurone disease. Her weakness slowly progressed and eventually she died of respiratory failure. No other relative was known to suffer from a similar disease, although no special enquiry had been made into her family history.

Necropsy Findings (Dr J Rivett, Stoke Mandeville Hospital, Aylesbury)

In the general necropsy the cause of death was shown to be bronchopneumonia. The brain was macroscopically normal. Histologically in the brain stem there was bilateral pyramidal tract degeneration evident in the medulla but not detectable in the pons or the midbrain. The spinal cord was moderately atrophied with wasting of the anterior spinal nerve roots. Histological sections of many cord segments showed tract degenerations affecting the direct and indirect corticospinal tracts, the gracile and cuneate fasciculi of the posterior columns and the anterior and posterior spino-cerebellar tracts (Figure 1). The corticospinal tract degeneration was moderate in the indirect (crossed) tract and slight in the direct (uncrossed) tract. This tract degeneration clearly increased caudally. In the grey matter of the spinal cord (Figures 2 and 3) there were conspicuous changes in Clarke's column (Figure 2) and in the anterior horn (Figure 3). The neurone cells bodies of Clarke's column were virtually absent and these nuclei could only be identified by their shape as areas of astrocytic fibrous gliosis (Figure 2). No inclusion

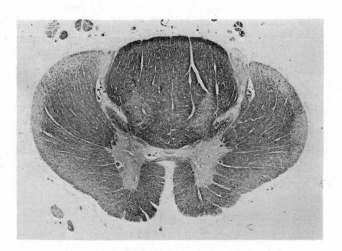

Figure 1. Photomicrograph of myelin-stained transverse section of spinal cord at T11 segmental level. There is degeneration of the anterior and posterior spinocerebellar tracts, of the cortico-spinal tracts and of the posterior columns. Note the shape of the tract degeneration in the cuneate fasciculi of the posterior columns. Weil x 12 (reduced for publication)

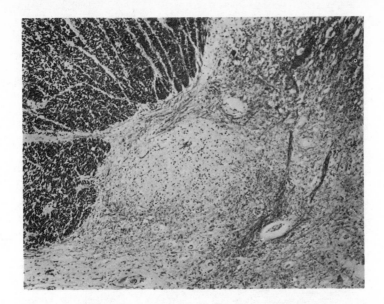

Figure 2. Photomicrograph of transverse section of spinal cord at T10 segmental level. The rounded nucleus dorsalis (Clarke's column) is empty of neurones and seen only as a cluster of astrocytes. Luxol blue/cresyl violet, x 90 (reduced for publication)

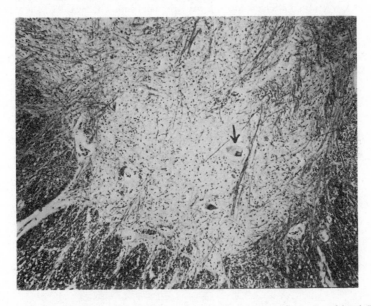

Figure 3. Photomicrograph of transverse section of spinal cord at S2 segmental level. The picture shows the right anterior horn in which only two large neurones remain. The one indicated by the arrow shows distension of the cytoplasm and displacement of the nucleus. Luxol blue/cresyl violet, x 90 (reduced for publication)

105

material could be seen in the cytoplasm of any of the cells in the region of Clarke's column presumably because of the virtual absence of neurones. The anterior horns were severely depleted of neurone cell bodies and were affected

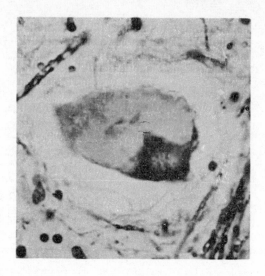

Figure 4. Detail at high magnification of abnormal motor neurone cell body seen in Figure 3. The nucleus has been displaced at the lower right hand corner of the cell by the abnormal material in the cytoplasm. Luxol blue/cresyl violet, x 600 (reduced for publication)

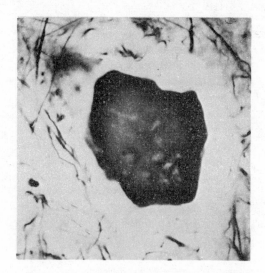

Figure 5. Same neurone cell body as in Figure 4 but stained with a silver technique. The abnormal material is feebly argyrophilic. Holmes x 600 (reduced for publication)

by gliosis. The striking finding was that the few surviving anterior horn motor neurones were frequently swollen by the presence of abnormal intracytoplasmic inclusion material (Figures 3, 4 and 5). These altered cell bodies were found at all levels of the spinal cord but were most readily seen in the cervical enlargement and in the lumbosacral region. They were not found in the motor nuclei of the brain stem. A typically abnormal perikaryon contained this poorly-stained material which enlarged the cell and displaced the nucleus and former cytoplasm in the periphery (Figure 4). The material was usually present as one mass but occasionally two or more separate aggregates were present. A vacuolar appearance within this material was probably due to the presence of surviving cytoplasm. The abnormal material stained faintly with eosin but did not stain with cresyl violet in the Nissl preparations. With the Holmes silver stain (Figure 5) and with von Braunmühl's method the material was moderately argyrophilic. No fine structure could be made out with these silver techniques, and there was no resemblance to the neurofibrillary tangle of Alzheimer's disease. The material was not doubly refractile. The anterior spinal nerve roots were markedly atrophied and fibrotic at all segmental levels but the posterior nerve roots appeared normal. Sections of skeletal muscles showed groups of atrophied muscle fibres giving a pattern suggestive of chronic denervation.

Electron Microscopy (Figures 6–9)

Several blocks of tissue from the anterior horns of the formalin-fixed spinal cord were post-fixed in buffered osmium tetroxide, embedded in araldite and thick sections were cut and examined. Scrutiny of these thick sections enabled a choice of blocks containing an anterior horn cell with inclusion material and these selected blocks were further trimmed for ultra-thin section cutting. By this means sections were cut from several neurone cell bodies containing intracytoplasmic inclusion material. At low magnifications a perikaryon containing the abnormal material was readily recognised (Figure 6). The cell body was moderately swollen and the nucleus and some surviving cytoplasma was displaced to one corner of the cell. The remaining cytoplasm was compressed into a thin peripheral rim in the cell except for traces of cytoplasm inside the abnormal material. There was no limiting membrane between the abnormal material and the displaced cytoplasm but at the interface between the two regions a zone of lipofuscin was commonly present (Figures 7 and 8). At higher magnifications (Figure 9) the abnormal material was seen to be made up of filaments. These were unbranching filaments whose diameter was of the order of 10 nanometres (nm). The filaments lacked any obvious orientation and groups were often seen transversely cut, adjacent to filaments orientated longitudinally (Figure 9). Scattered among the masses of filaments were areas of amorphous electron dense material which were probably remains of the normal cytoplasm of the cell. The nature of these abnormal filaments was

107

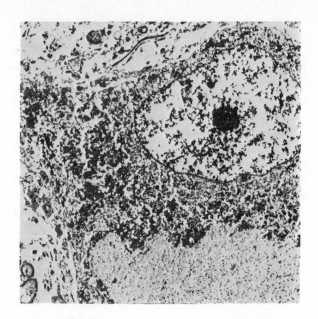

Figure 6. Electron micrograph of ultra-thin section of a neurone cell body from the left anterior horn of C8 spinal cord segment. The nucleus and cytoplasm have been displaced to the periphery of the cell (upper part of picture) by the material seen below. Compare with Figure 4. Formalin fixation, post-fixation in osmium (1% Caulfield's). Stained with 2% uranyl acetate and lead citrate. x 4600 (reduced for publication)

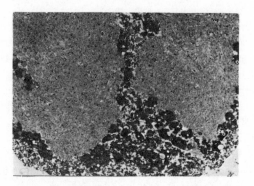

Figure 7. Electron micrograph of ultra-thin section of a neurone cell body from the right anterior horn of C1 spinal cord segment. Two masses of abnormal material are separated by surviving cytoplasm and lipofuscin material. Note the island of lipofuscin (left) within the abnormal material. Preparative details as for Figure 6. x 4600 (reduced for publication)

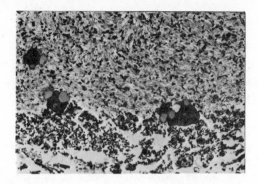

Figure 8. Electron micrograph of ultra-thin section of a neurone cell body from the left anterior horn of C8 spinal cord segment. At this higher magnification the material is seen to be made up of filaments seen longitudinally or cut in cross section (centre). Note the lipofuscin within the material (top left) and (below) at the edge between the material and the surviving cytoplasm. Preparative details as for Figure 6 x 7000 (reduced for publication)

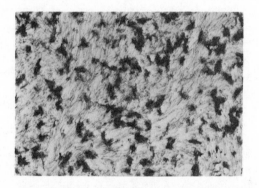

Figure 9. Electron micrograph at high magnification of material seen in Figures 6, 7 and 8. Filaments of approximately 10 nm are seen longitudinally and (centre) cut in transverse section. The amorphous dense material is probably surviving cytoplasm. Preparative detail as for Figure 6. x 20,000 (reduced for publication)

clearly of great interest and a comparison was made with the findings reported by Schochet et al (1969). Dr SS Schochet, then of the University of Iowa, kindly made available ultrathin sections of his material and comparable electron micrographs were successively obtained on the two cases. This direct comparison conclusively showed the two examples of abnormal filaments to be of the same size and structure.

DISCUSSION

The findings of abnormally disposed masses of filaments in the neurones of various neurological diseases has focused attention again on the ultrastructure

109

of the normal neurofilament. Peters et al (1970) reviewed ultrastructural observations on microtubules and neurofilaments found in normal mammalian neurones. The microtubule is a long tubular element 20—26 nm in diameter. On transverse section it appears as a circle with a dense wall some 6 nm thick. The normal filament is about 10 nm in diameter and is also tubular. On transverse section, if well seen, it appears as a round structure with an outer dense layer 3 nm thick surrounding a lighter core.

We are now in a position to summarise the observations concerning abnormal neurofibrillary material in the neurones of cases of neurological diseases and to relate the observations to the normal anatomical neurotubule or neurofibril. The neurofilaments described in the case referred to here are of a similar size to normal neurofilaments. The abnormal appearance in the neurones is due to excessive numbers of the filaments and also to their tangled form which results in the light microscopical appearance of hyaline intracytoplasmic material. The abnormality is similar to that found in other cases of motor neurone disease. The experimentally induced neurofibrillary change described earlier is also formed from an accumulation of neurofilaments of normal size and form. We have therefore a group of conditions, including motor neurone disease, various toxic and metabolic human diseases and various experimental neuronal degeneration, in which there is an extensive abnormal production in the neurone cell body of neurofilaments which are relatively normal in size and morphology. The significance of this finding is as yet uncertain but it may indicate an attempt of the neurone cell body to repair damage to the axon. It is interesting that in the case described here the long tract degeneration had the feature that the part of the axon remote from the cell body was more affected than the part near the cell body.

The abnormal filaments of Alzheimer's disease which are also found in the inherited neurological disease of Guam Island, in Pick's disease, and in post-encephalitic Parkinsonism appear quite different from the neurofibrillary pathology in motor neurone disease. In Alzheimer's disease we are dealing with a large diameter filament of the order of size of the normal neurotubule. The nature of this abnormal filament, which morphologically is distinctive because of regular constrictions, is controversial but this type of filament has not been seen in motor neurone disease.

Acknowledgment

The author acknowledges with gratitude the permission of Elsevier, North Holland Biomedical press BV to reproduce illustrations and text that appeared in the report by Hughes and Jerrome (1971).

References

Carpenter, S (1968) *Neurology (Minneapolis), 18,* 841
Engel, WK, Kurland, LT and Klatzo, I (1959) *Brain, 82,* 203

Hirano, A, Kurland, LT and Sayre, GP (1967) *Archives of Neurology (Chicago)*, *16*, 232

Hirano, A, Malamud, N, Elizan, TS and Kurland, LT (1966) *Archives of Neurology (Chicago)*, *15*, 35

Hughes, JT and Jerrome, D (1971) *Journal of the Neurological Sciences, 13*, 389

Kidd, M (1963) *Nature (London), 197*, 192

Klatzo, I, Wisniewski, H and Streicher, E (1965) *Journal of Neuropathology and Experimental Neurology, 24*, 187

Kurland, LT and Mulder, DW (1955) *Neurology (Minneapolis), 5*, 182 and 249

Peters, A, Palay, SL and Webster, H deF (1970) *The Fine Structure of the Nervous System.* Harper and Row, New York

Schochet, SS, Lampert, PW and Lindenberg, R (1968) *Acta Neuropathologica (Berlin), 11*, 330

Schochet, SS, Hardman, JM, Ladewig, PP and Earle, KM (1969) *Archives of Neurology (Chicago), 20*, 548

Terry, RD (1963) *Journal of Neuropathology and Experimental Neurology, 22*, 629

Wisniewski, H, Shelanski, ML and Terry, RD (1968) *Journal of Cell Biology, 38*, 224

Wisniewski, H, Terry, RD and Hirano, A (1970) *Journal of Neuropathology and Experimental Neurology, 29*, 163

CHAPTER ELEVEN

INTERPRETATION OF ELECTROMYOGRAPHICAL DATA IN SPINAL MUSCULAR ATROPHY

John E Desmedt and S Borenstein

The study of electrical activity of muscle discloses a number of characteristic changes in patients with spinal muscular atrophy. Electromyography (EMG) with the concentric needle electrode discloses both abnormal activities of muscle fibre (fibrillation potentials) and of motor units (fasciculation potentials) in relaxed muscle, and also marked changes in the motor unit potentials (MUPs) elicited by slight voluntary contraction. The latter MUP changes involve primarily increased duration and increased voltage which can considerably exceed the size of the potentials recorded in normal muscle, even at maximal contraction (Kugelberg, 1949; Buchthal, 1957, 1962; Lambert, 1969). In patients with slowly progressive spinal atrophy of the Kugelberg-Welander type, such increases in voltage of the MUPs are particularly striking since they can reach 20 mV, whereas the upper limit of the normal range is about 3 mV. The total duration of MUPs can easily be doubled, thus bringing mean duration of MUPs from about 10 msec to 15 or even 20 msec (Figure 1). These changes are more marked in proximal muscles than in distal muscle in patients with the Kugelberg-Welander syndrome and this obviously relates to the clinically observed distribution of muscle involvement. When the patient contracts muscle maximally, the number of different motor units which can be recorded at any one muscle site is much reduced, which reflects the small density of motor units resulting from loss of motoneurones.

The increased size of MUPs in spinal atrophy has been related by Wohlfart (1958) to collateral sprouting of healthy motor axons in the partially denervated muscles, and to reinnervation of denervated muscle fibres which have lost their original motor axon. This phenomenon considerably enlarges the size of the remaining motor units, and it concomitantly reduces the number of denervated muscle fibres, and thus also the incidence of spontaneous fibrillation potentials. The collateral reinnervation also contributes to delay and reduces atrophy and paresis which, at least before the late stages of the disease, are not proportional to the actual loss of motoneurones innervating the muscles considered.

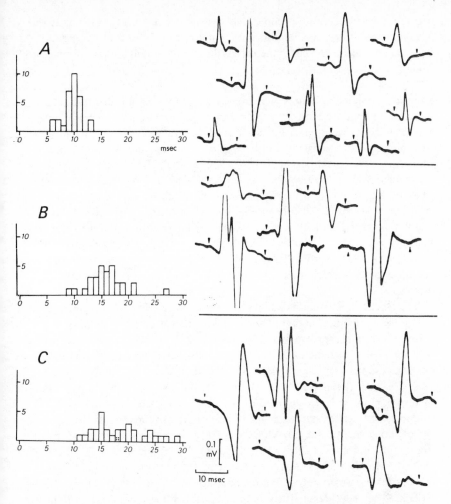

Figure 1. Histograms of total duration of different motor unit potentials on the left side. Abscissa, duration in msec. Ordinate, number of potentials measured (at least 5 samples of any MUP compared for consistent estimation of duration). Sample records of MUPs on the right side. A = normal subject of 20 years, adductor pollicis muscle. B and C = patient of 31 years with typical Kugelberg-Welander syndrome. Data for the adductor pollicis (B) and for the brachial biceps (C). The case in stipple indicates a polyphasic potential (more than 4 phases crossing the base line). Notice the more marked increases of duration and size in the proximal muscle in C (from Desmedt, 1967).

Thus, in a slowly progressive Kugelberg-Welander syndrome, MUPs become very large while spontaneous fibrillations can be scarce or even absent. On the other hand, in rapidly advancing amyotrophic lateral sclerosis, the increase in size of the MUPs is less important because collateral reinnervation by motor axons remaining healthy at any one time can only proceed for a limited period

113

before these axons in turn become involved and disintegrate. In such cases the collateral sprouting is unable to maintain innervation of most of the muscle fibres in the muscle and spontaneous fibrillation potentials are found more profusely.

So-called myopathic features in neurogenic atrophy Histological studies have shown, in the muscle biopsies of long-standing cases with neurogenic atrophy, a number of changes such as internal nuclei, variation in fibre size, focal necrosis, which had been considered rather typical of myopathic diseases (Pearce & Harriman, 1966; Drachman et al, 1967; Munsat et al, 1969; Mumenthaler, 1970; Mastaglia & Walton, 1971; Achari & Anderson, 1974). These features are now considered to result from the extensive metabolic changes associated mainly with cycles of denervation and collateral reinnervation of muscle fibres in those muscles undergoing slowly progressive partial denervation. It is also recognised that such concurrence of various histological features previously thought to characterise either neuropathic or myopathic disease processes may result in a confusing picture which limits the diagnostic usefulness of muscle biopsy in some patients.

The recent extensive use of EMG as a diagnostic aid in problem patients has also raised difficulties. In myopathic diseases, such as muscular dystrophy, motor units undergo a progressive loss of muscle fibres so that the potentials recorded with a concentric needle electrode present a characteristic reduction in both total duration and voltage (Kugelberg, 1949; Buchthal, 1957; Buchthal & Rosenfalck, 1963; Desmedt & Emeryk, 1968; Desmedt & Borenstein, 1976). In patients with spinal atrophy, the close observation of muscle potentials activated by slight voluntary contraction has occasionally disclosed a mixture of enlarged MUPs and of rather small potentials which resembled those expected in musclar dystrophy (cf Humphrey & Shy, 1962; Amick et al, 1966; Hausmanowa-Petrusewicz et al, 1968). When using EMG for identifying the neuropathic or myopathic nature of a disease process such mixed patterns have proved misleading and the EMG has been considered either as non-diagnostic or as conflicting with muscle biopsy data (Black et al, 1974).

We have carried out a detailed analysis of MUPs in several patients with neurogenic atrophy, by recording with a standard concentric needle electrode which was carefully positioned in different sites within the territory of chosen motor units. The potentials have been tape-recorded so that they could be played back for further study with the 'coherent EMG' display whereby a window-trigger electronic circuit enables the potential to start the oscilloscope sweeps and a digital delay line of 5 msec allows the initial part of the same potential to be displayed on the second beam of the oscilloscope (Borenstein and Desmedt, 1973; Desmedt & Borenstein, 1973, 1976).

When looking at free-running sweeps, as routinely done in standard EMG, it is common to observe so-called mixed patterns including both large MUPs of the

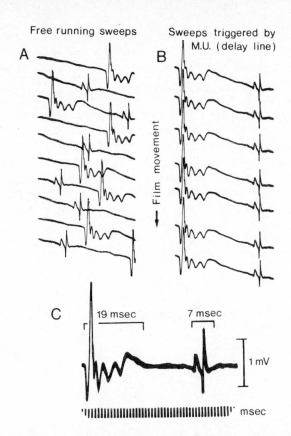

Figure 2. Male patient of 57 years with a typical spinal muscular atrophy of the Kugelberg-Welander type, with a slow progression since the age of 11 years. The patient has not been able to walk since the age of 14 years. Muscle paresis with proximal predominance in the lower limbs, and also in the upper limbs, with diffuse fasciculations and absent tendon reflexes. No sensory signs. Electromyograms recorded with a concentric electrode in the brachial biceps muscle (Temperature of the muscle 35°C). A = free running oscilloscope sweeps. B = sweeps triggered by the same motor unit, disclosing a consistent 'linked potential'. C = same motor unit potential displayed by superimposing a dozen different sweeps. The total duration of the MUP and of the 'linked potential' are indicated

type expected in spinal atrophy and small and brief potentials which look very much like the MUPs found in advanced muscular dystrophy (Figure 2A). However when the same data are observed in a 'coherent EMG' display, it becomes obvious that the smaller potential is not an independent MUP, but is actually a 'linked potential' discharging with a rather consistent time delay after the main MUP (Figure 2B). Various controls convinced us that these 'linked potentials' are not just repetitive discharges of a part of the main MUP, since their size and shape can be changed independently by slight movements of the recording electrode. Furthermore the 'linked potentials' cannot be interpreted as a reflex

115

discharge because they occur at a variety of latencies, up to 80 msec, in different MUPs: there are indeed no preferred latencies with respect to the main MUP when muscles at different distances from the spinal cord are studied (Desmedt & Borenstein, 1973, 1976).

'Linked potentials' have been consistently found in spinal atrophy and also in patients with partial denervation due to traumatic lesions of peripheral nerves (Borenstein & Desmedt, 1973). They are interpreted as the discharge of muscle fibres which have been collaterally reinnervated by sprouts from a motor axon. The delay between the main MUP and the 'linked potential' can be related to slow conduction in a long collateral sprout of small diameter, and perhaps also to a longer conduction time in the corresponding muscle fibres between the newly formed endplate and the level of the recording electrode. As shown by

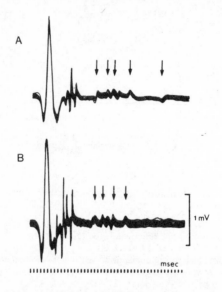

Figure 3. Female patient of 12 years with a typical spinal muscular atrophy of the Kugelberg-Welander type since the age of 5 years. Proximal paresis and atrophy of the four limbs (more marked in the lower limbs), with a few diffuse fasciculations and absent tendon reflexes. No sensory signs. The patient was still able to walk, but with some difficulties. Two different motor unit potentials are illustrated and their consistent wave forms shown by superimposing a dozen successive sweeps. The 'linked potentials' are indicated by arrows. They are preceded by 'early linked potentials'. Muscle temperature 35°C. (From Borenstein & Desmedt, 1973).

Figure 3, for a patient with Kugelberg-Welander syndrome, quite a few 'linked potentials' can be seen after the main MUP, and one can even distinguish between late (arrows) and early 'linked potentials', which simply imply different delays for activation of the action potential in the different, collaterally reinnervated, muscle fibres. The increased size and duration of the main MUP would then be viewed as resulting from collaterally innervated muscle fibres which are triggered with rather short delays so that they are integrated into the relatively smooth wave form of the main MUP.

When muscle fibres are collaterally reinnervated, the neuromuscular transmission process presents initially a small safety factor which results in random variations over about 2 msec of the latency of the 'linked potential' and even in occasional blockings, as illustrated for the linked potentials labelled 2 and 3 in Figure 4. In these instances, the latency is not absolutely stable but presents

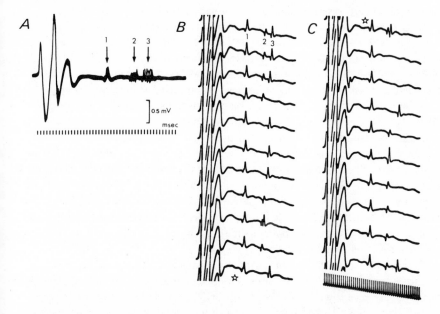

Figure 4. Same patient as in Figure 2. Another motor unit potential recorded by a concentric needle electrode in the brachial biceps. A = superimposed sweeps showing three different 'linked potentials' after the large main motor unit potential. The 'linked potentials' labelled 2 and 3 show slightly variable latency. The same potentials are displayed in B and C (continuous record) on moving photographic film. The amplification used does not allow seeing the full magnitude of the main MUP. 'Linked potential' No.1 has a stable latency, whereas 'linked potentials' Nos.2 and 3 present random variations in their latencies and occasional blockings. They are easily identified by their different wave forms. (From Borenstein and Desmedt, 1973)

variations about a mean value which is characteristic for the component considered. As a rule, the safety factor for neuromuscular transmission improves with time, and the latency of 'linked potentials' become then quite stable while blockings no longer occur, as shown from the consistent superimposition of the 'linked potentials', both early and late, in Figure 3. The above interpretation is supported from observations on 'linked potentials' developing after a partial traumatic nerve lesion, the date of which is known. The slight variations of the latencies of 'linked potentials' about a mean value are then observed in the early stages after

117

the lesion only (Borenstein & Desmedt, 1973).

Diagnostic uses of EMG in spinal atrophy The EMG is of great value to identify
the disease at early stages when the clinical picture is incomplete or doubtful.

When fasciculations are not visible through the skin in obese patients, or in
infants (where subcutaneous fat obscures the muscle contour) with suspected
Werdnig-Hoffmann disease, or in patients with suspected Kugelberg-Welander
syndrome (where fasciculations are generally rare), the EMG can help to demonstrate spontaneous fasciculations in the deeper parts of the limb muscles.

EMG examination is also quite helpful in diagnosing the Kugelberg-Welander
syndrome which has often been confused with Duchenne muscular dystrophy
since it affects predominantly the proximal muscles of the limbs. The EMG will
show large size MUPs and reduced numbers of MUPs at maximum contraction.
The small potentials which may be present in the record should be properly
identified as 'linked potentials' rather than as spurious so-called 'myopathic'
MUPs. It must be stressed that the failure to record spontaneous fibrillation
potentials is definitely not against a diagnosis of Kugelberg-Welander syndrome
since this simply reflects in these patients the efficiency of the collateral reinnervation process at early stages of the disease. On the other hand it must be stressed
that spontaneous fibrillations are quite consistently recorded (contrary to earlier
beliefs) in muscles of patients with myopathies and particularly in Duchenne
muscular dystrophy (Desmedt & Borenstein, 1975, 1976). Thus the presence of
spontaneous fibrillations in a patient should no longer be considered as foolproof
evidence for a neuropathic disorder.

There are occasionally patients with abundant fasciculations as the presenting
symptom and who disclose virtually no weakness or atrophy on clinical examination. We have recently seen such a patient of 56 years whose diagnosis of amyotrophic lateral sclerosis had been overlooked by several competent neurologists,
but who was found to present typically enlarged MUPs in the limbs, thus eviden-
cing an active process of denervation and collateral reinnervation. On the other
hand, if a person with spontaneous fasciculations presents an EMG with no
abnormal MUPs, this provides useful evidence for a diagnosis of benign fasciculations and reassurance for the patient.

The abnormal MUPs found in a systematic EMG examination can also serve to
demonstrate a wider distribution in limb muscles of a process which may have
appeared to be localised on clinical examination: this is helpful in providing evidence against a localised nerve lesion (eg entrapment) and in favour of a more
generalised neuropathic disorder.

Summary

The electromyographical (EMG) features of neurogenic atrophy are reviewed
critically in order to identify the mechanisms underlying the changes in motor

118

unit potential (MUP) wave form, voltage and duration. The occurrence of 'linked potentials' which can follow the main MUP by up to 80 msec, in spinal atrophy is emphasised because they provide useful evidence concerning collateral reinnervation of denervated muscle fibres and the dynamic changes of the motor unit. These 'linked potentials' have been misinterpreted as 'myopathic' potentials, leading to a confused interpretation of routine EMG data. It is also shown that fibrillation potentials can be quite rare in slowly progressive spinal atrophy, for example, Kugelberg-Welander syndrome, because of the efficiency of collateral reinnervation. On the other hand spontaneous fibrillation potentials are now recognised as a common finding in myopathies and particularly in Duchenne muscular dystrophy. The inadequate interpretation of fibrillation potentials in the neuromuscular diseases has no doubt also contributed to errors in EMG diagnosis. Typical examples of the uses of EMG in the diagnosis of neuropathic lesions are discussed.

Acknowledgments

The research reported has been supported in part by the Muscular Dystrophy Association of America, the Fonds de la Recherche Scientifique Médicale and the Fonds National de la Recherche Scientifique.

References

Achari, AN and Anderson, S (1974) *Neurology (Minneap), 24,* 477

Adams, RD, Denny-Brown, D and Pearson, CM (1962) *Diseases of Muscle. A Study in Pathology.* Hoeber, New York

Amick, LD, Smith, HL and Johnson, WW (1966) *Acta neurologica Scandinavica, 42,* 275

Black, JT, Bhatt, GP, DeJesus, PV, Schotland, DL and Rowland, LP (1974) *Journal of Neurological Science, 21,* 59

Borenstein, S and Desmedt, JE (1973) In *New Developments in Electromyography and Clinical Neurophysiology.* (Ed) JE Desmedt. Karger, Basel. Page 130

Buchthal, F (1957) *An Introduction to Electromyography.* Gylendal, Copenhagen

Buchthal, F (1962) *World Neurology, 3,* 16

Buchthal, F and Rosenfalck, P (1963) In *Muscular Dystrophy in Man and Animals.* (Ed) GH Bourne and MN Golarz. Karger, Basel. Page 193

Desmedt, JE (1967) *Bulletin de l'Académie royale de médecine de Belgique, VIIe serie, 7,* 701

Desmedt, JE and Emeryk, B (1968) *American Journal of Medicine, 45,* 853

Desmedt, JE and Borenstein, S (1973) *Nature (London), 246,* 500

Desmedt, JE and Borenstein, S (1975) *Nature (London), 258,* 531

Desmedt, JE and Borenstein, S (1976) *Archives of Neurology (Chicago), 33,* 642

Drachman, DB, Murphy, SR, Nigam, MP and Hills, JR (1967) *Archives of Neurology (Chicago), 16,* 14

Hausmanova-Petrusewicz, Emeryk, B, Wasowicz, B and Kopec, A (1967)

Electromyography, 7, 203

Humphrey, JG and Shy, GM (1962) *Archives of Neurology (Chicago), 6,* 339

Kugelberg, E (1949) *Journal of Neurology, Neurosurgery and Psychiatry, 12,* 129

Lambert, EH (1969) In *Motor Neuron Diseases.* (Ed) FH Norris and LT Kurland. Grune and Stratton, New York. Page 135

Mastaglia, FL and Walton, JN (1971) *Journal of Neurological Science, 12,* 15

Mumenthaler, M (1970) In *Muscle Disease.* (Ed) JN Walton, N Canal and G Scarlato. Abstracts of paper presented at the International Congress on Muscle Diseases, Milan 1969. International Congress Series No 186. Excerpta Medica, Amsterdam. Page 585

Munsat, TL, Woods, R, Fooler, W and Pearson, CM (1969) *Brain, 92,* 9

Pearce, J and Harriman, DGF (1966) *Journal of Neurology, Neurosurgery and Psychiatry, 29,* 509

Wohlfart, G (1958) *Neurology (Minneapolis), 8,* 175

CHAPTER TWELVE

SLOW VIRUSES AND MOTOR NEURONE DISEASE

W B Matthews

The recent increased awareness of the role of viruses and of other less well characterised transmissible agents in the causation of chronic or relapsing disease of the nervous system has naturally led to renewed attempts to demonstrate a viral origin of motor neurone disease. All such attempts have so far proved unsuccessful and although I have no remarkable original observations to communicate, there are, a few marginal advances that at least indicate possible lines of further investigation.

The first of these dates back to the pandemic of encephalitis lethargica after the first world war. Over 20 years ago, with the late Dr Greenfield I reviewed the possible connection between encephalitis or recognisable post-encephalitic syndromes and motor neurone disease (Greenfield and Matthews, 1954). It was never possible to produce figures to demonstrate that the association was anything more than coincidental, but we considered a causal connection probable. There is considerable evidence that a condition clinically indistinguishable from motor neurone disease in its various forms could occur many years after an attack of encephalitis, usually long preceded by well recognised post-encephalitic symptoms. In my own case in whom the encephalitis could be dated, parkinson-ism with oculogyric crises and torticollis developed after 10 years and motor neurone disease of the amyotrophic lateral sclerosis type after a further 12 years. In my second case, no attack of encephalitis could be recognised, but very slowly developing parkinsonism was also accompanied by oculogyric crises. Motor neurone disease of the progressive muscular atrophy type developed 25 years later and was fatal within 18 months.

In most reported cases amyotrophy has begun in the upper limbs, but bulbar palsy can also be the presenting feature. In our case where an autopsy was obtained, Dr Greenfield did not find neuro-fibrillary changes in the spinal cord

121

and there was no long tract degeneration. The pathogenesis of the anterior horn cell degeneration could not be established.

The only possible relevance in this ancient history is the recent demonstration by Gamboa et al (1974) of intranuclear antigen, staining with fluorescent antibodies to two neurotropic strains of influenza A in the midbrain and hypothalamus of the six cases of post-encephalitic parkinsonism they examined. Antigen was not present in the brain in idiopathic Parkinson's disease. Virologists find it puzzling that a positive reaction was not obtained with all strains of influenza A virus, but the evidence is sufficiently striking and has neither been confirmed nor refuted. Although a positive result is unlikely, an attempt should certainly be made to detect influenza antigen in cases of sporadic motor neurone disease.

Attempts to incriminate other identified viruses have also been based on clinical associations. Quick (1969) reported the remarkable finding that five of his 15 cases had sustained an attack of mumps in adult life, but this was not confirmed by Lehrich et al (1974) who were also unable to demonstrate neutralising antibodies to mumps in 27 cases. The evidence for an association of motor neurone disease with a previous attack of paralytic poliomyelitis is much stronger, although I do not believe it has ever been strong enough to convince Dr Kurland. There have been various reports of progressive muscular wasting developing many years after paralytic poliomyelitis and, indeed, I imagine that every experienced neurologist has seen this on a number of occasions. From personal experience, this is certainly not the belated effect on locomotion of long existing paralysis, and is a progressive disease affecting areas not known to have been involved in the acute paralysis. The incidence of paralytic polio in patients diagnosed as motor neurone disease has been variously estimated as 10% (Zilkha, 1962), 5% (Norris et al, 1975), and 2.5% (Poskanzer et al, 1969). The relevance of these surprisingly high figures must depend on whether the progressive disorder that these patients undoubtedly develop is identical with sporadic motor neurone disease. Mulder et al (1972) concluded that it was not, basing this conclusion on the relatively slow progression of the disease and the comparative rarity of upper motor neurone signs. Others have commented on the benign course of the disease (Campbell et al, 1969) but this is certainly not invariable (Norris et al, 1975), nor is a prolonged course incompatible with the classical form of motor neurone disease, occurring in approximately 10% of cases (Vejjajiva et al, 1967). I have not found a report of a case examined histologically, although it is doubtful whether such an examination would be illuminating.

It has been variously postulated that anterior horn cells damaged in the original attack of poliomyelitis are subject to premature abiotrophy or that persistent poliovirus causes progressive disease ten or more years later. There is so far no immunological evidence for this latter theory as neither serum neutralising (Lehrich et al, 1974) nor complement fixation (Cremer et al, 1973) antibodies to poliovirus are increased above control values. The CSF does not seem to have been examined for antibodies. No virus has been demonstrated by immunofluorescent antibody staining of tissue cultures from classical motor neurone disease (Cremer et al, 1973).

Following the success in transmitting Creutzfeldt-Jakob disease (CJD) to laboratory animals (Gibbs et al, 1968) motor neurone disease was naturally high on the list of diseases possibly in the same category. Muscular wasting, fasciculation and anterior horn cell loss may all occur in CJD and the spongy degeneration, so common in this disease, has been reported in motor neurone disease (Brownell et al, 1970) although I am not certain that in at least one of these cases the diagnosis was not that of CJD. This only serves to emphasise the points of resemblance between the two conditions. Lower motor neurone involvement is comparatively rare in the transmissible form of CJD but does occur (Roos et al, 1973). Classical motor neurone disease has not been transmitted in this way (Gibbs and Gajdusek, 1972). Negative results of transmission experiments with possible slow viruses are difficult to interpret with any finality in view of the 8½ years needed for successful transmission of kuru to the rhesus monkey (Gajdusek and Gibbs, 1972). The Russian claim to have transmitted motor neurone disease to monkeys could not be confirmed using identical material, nor could the histological changes reported in the animals be identified (Brody et al, 1965).

There have been surprisingly few reports of 'virus-like particles' in motor neurone disease. A major difficulty with such findings in chronic neurological disease is to establish whether the presumed viruses are related to the pathological process or are merely harmless occupants or terminal invaders of the nervous system. Bunina (cited by Hirano et al, 1965) reported eosinophilic inclusions in affected anterior horn cells. Using EM, Sun et al (1975) found inclusion bodies, possibly in neurones, in a case of classical motor neurone disease. These were not identified by light microscopy and the authors considered that they resembled Lafora bodies and were of metabolic origin. Norris et al (1975) described a unique case of a man with multiple recurrent attacks of lymphocytic meningitis of unknown cause and, eventually, motor neurone disease. At autopsy interwoven serpentine tubules were found within neurones. These were thought to resemble myxovirus but none could be recovered from tissue culture. Oshiro et al (1976) recently described crystalline arrays of presumed virus particles in the muscles of a patient with typical motor neurone disease, but again, attempts to identify the agent were unsuccessful.

These largely negative results may, of course, mean that transmissible agents are not involved in the pathogenesis of motor neurone disease but may be merely a reflection of inadequate technique.

References

Brody, JA, Hadlow, WJ, Hotchin, J, Johnson, RT, Kopiowski, H and Kurland, LT (1965) *Science, 147,* 1114

Brownell, B, Oppenheimer, DR and Hughes, JT (1970) *Neurosurgery and Psychiatry, 33,* 338

Campbell, AMG, Williams, ER and Pearce, J (1969) *Neurology (Minneapolis), 19,* 1101

Cremer, NE, Oshiro, LS, Norris, FH and Lennette, EH (1973) *Archives of Neurology, 29,* 331

Gajdusek, DC and Gibbs, CJ (1972) *Nature, 240,* 351

Gamboa, ET, Wolf, A, Yahr, MD, Harter, DH, Duffy, PE, Barden, H and Hus, KC (1974) *Archives of Neurology, 31,* 228

Gibbs, CJ and Gajdusek, DC (1972) *Journal of Clinical Pathology, 25 (Suppt.6) (Royal College of Pathologists),* 132

Gibbs, CJ, Gajdusek, DC, Asher, DM, Alpers, MP, Beck, E, Daniel, PM and Matthews, WB (1968) *Science, 161,* 388

Greenfield, JG and Matthews, WB (1954) *Neurosurgery and Psychiatry, 17,* 50

Hirano, A, Malamud, N, Kurland, LT and Zimmerman, HM (1965) In *Motor Neurone Diseases.* (Ed) FH Norris and LT Kurland. Grune and Stratton, New York. Page 51

Lehrich, JR, Oger, J and Arnason, BGW (1974) *Journal of the Neurological Sciences, 23,* 537

Mulder, DW, Rosenblum, RA and Layton, DD (1972) *Mayo Clinic Proceedings, 47,* 756

Norris, FH, Aguilar, MJ, Colton, RP, Oldstone, MBA and Cremer, NE (1975) *Journal of Neuropathology and Experimental Neurology, 34,* 133

Oshiro, LS, Cremer, NE, Norris, FH and Lennette, EH (1976) *Neurology (Minneapolis), 26,* 57

Poskanzer, DC, Cantor, HM and Caplan, GS (1969) In *Motor Neurone Diseases.* (Ed) FH Norris and LT Kurland. Grune and Stratton, New York. Page 286

Quick, DT (1969) In *Motor Neurone Diseases.* (Ed) FH Norris and LT Kurland. Grune and Stratton, New York. Page 189

Roos, R, Gajdusek, DC and Gibbs, CJ (1973) *Brain, 96,* 1

Sun, CN, Araoz, C, Lucas, G, Morgan, PN and White, HJ (1975) *Annals of Clinical and Laboratory Science, 5,* 38

Vejjajiva, A, Foster, JB and Miller, H (1967) *Journal of the Neurological Sciences, 4,* 299

Zilkha, KJ (1962) *Proceedings of the Royal Society of Medicine, 55,* 1028

CHAPTER THIRTEEN

ALPHA-ADRENOCEPTOR BLOCKING AGENTS IN THE TREATMENT OF SPASTICITY

Christopher de Bois White and Alan Richens

The work presented in this chapter was stimulated by a chance observation that the alpha-adrenoceptor blocking agent, thymoxamine, markedly depressed triceps surae tendon jerk responses in human volunteers who received the drug intravenously (Figure 1). This observation was made during a study of the effects of β-adrenoceptor blocking agents on the central nervous system; these latter compounds, however, failed to influence the tendon jerk response, in contrast to thymoxamine. A further study indicated that methylamphetamine, an indirectly-acting sympathomimetic drug, caused an increase in the amplitude of the tendon jerk response, suggesting that an a-adrenoceptor mechanism might be involved in the physiological regulation of this reflex pathway (Phillips, Richens and Shand, 1973).

A review of earlier neuropharmacological studies in animals revealed evidence which supported the role of monoamines in the regulation of reflex activity. The histochemical fluorescence studies of Dahlström and Fuxe (1965) demonstrated that, in every species of animal examined, noradrenergic bulbospinal tracts were present, apparently as the caudal projection of a diffusely projecting noradrena-line-containing neurone system, with cell bodies in the pons and medulla and terminations in many parts of the central nervous sytem. The finding of suitably placed catecholamine-containing cell bodies and tracts in the brain of the human foetus strongly suggests the presence of a similar noradrenergic system in man (Nobin and Bjorklund, 1972).

The perikarya of bulbospinal noradrenaline-containing neurones have been located in the ventromedial part of the lower medullary reticular formation (Dahlström and Fuxe, 1965). Their axons descend mainly in the anterior funiculi of the cord and were found to be small and unmyelinated. Numerous noradrenaline-containing nerve terminals were found in the ventral horn of the spinal cord, with dense distribution mainly in the areas containing a-motoneurone perikarya. The terminals made contact with small, medium-sized and large cell bodies and their processes. Some were in intimate contact with large motoneurones but it was

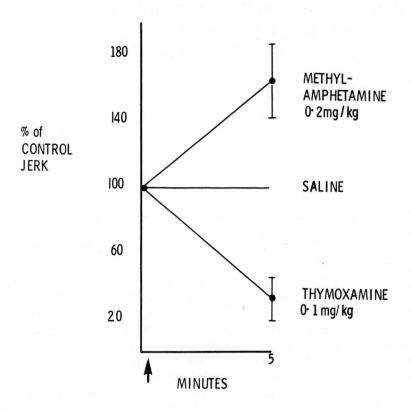

Figure 1   Effect of intravenous thymoxamine (0.1 mg/kg) and methylamphetamine (0.2 mg/kg) on triceps surae tendon jerk responses in six healthy volunteers. The bars represent one S.E.

not possible to determine whether they made contact with fusimotor neurones directly or not. The virtual disappearance of noradrenaline from the distal part of the spinal cord after transection confirmed its supraspinal origin (Anden et al, 1964). Electrical stimulation of tracts in the upper cervical region causes release of noradrenaline (Anden et al, 1965).

Experiments in which noradrenaline has been injected intravenously have produced conflicting results, presumably because this catecholamine does not readily enter the central nervous system from the vascular compartment. L-dopa is a precursor to dopamine and noradrenaline but differs from these two compounds in that it readily crosses the blood brain barrier, as evidenced by its effectiveness in treating patients with Parkinsonism. Experiments with this substance indicate that it produces a long latency, facilitatory effect on flexor reflexes, leading to an increase of both a-and γ-motoneurone output (Anden et al, 1966ab). In addition, the disposition of fusimotor neurone firing is altered by L-dopa. For flexor muscles in the lower limb, 'static' γ-motoneurones are activated while 'dynamic' γ-motoneurones are inhibited, whereas both types of motoneurone activity to extensor muscles are activated (Grillner, 1969). At the gross level, L-dopa activates bilaterally coordinated stepping activity, an effect which is also produced by amphetamine and methoxamine and reversed by alpha-adrenoceptor blockade in spinal dogs (Martin and Eades, 1967), and produced by intrathecal noradrenaline in intact cats (Dhawan and Sharma, 1970).

The question which arises from these studies is whether the effects of these indirectly-acting drugs are due to alpha-adrenoceptor stimulation or to some other mechanism. The non-involvement of a dopaminergic mechanism has been convincingly demonstrated by Anden et al (1970) by differentiating the effects of a series of neuroleptic agents on L-dopa induced changes in the corpus striatum and the spinal cord, and correlating them with the changes in dopamine and noradrenaline turnover produced by the drugs. The relative dopamine and noradrenaline blocking potencies of the drugs used in their experiments correlated with the findings of Janssen (1970). The results of blockade of other alpha-adrenoceptor agonists (Martin and Eades, 1967), dopamine beta-hydroxylase inhibition (Anden and Fuxe, 1971), and noradrenaline liberation (Fedina, Lundberg and Vyklicky, 1971) in spinal animals support the contention that alpha-adrenoceptor mechanisms alone can produce the described reflex changes. Ellaway and Pascoe (1968) measured γ-motoneurone discharges in spinal rabbit preparations while stimulating the cord below the transection, and administered drugs which both block and enhance noradrenergic activity. Their results also suggested that a polysynaptic noradrenergic pathway enhanced γ-motoneurone activity.

Of the many supraspinal influences on a- and γ-motoneurone activity, there are two important areas in which noradrenaline may be implicated, the cerebellar-vestibular system and the reticular formation, and these areas are known to exert a major control over segmental reflex activity. Classical decerebrate rigidity, which is produced by midbrain section at the level of the red nucleus, results from excessive neural drive emanating from the lateral vestibular nucleus and probably also from the large reticular neurones in the lower pons (Denny-Brown, 1966). It is dependent on fusimotor drive and is abolished by dorsal root section. Studies with chlorpromazine and other phenothiazines (Keary and Maxwell, 1967) and particularly thymoxamine and M and B 18706 (Maxwell and Sumpter, 1972; Maxwell, Read and Sumpter, 1974) have strongly suggested that alpha-adrenoceptor mechanisms are involved in the production of classical decerebrate rigidity, while they play no part after anterior cerebellar destruction (which converts to an a-motoneurone drive state in the decerebrate animal).

The site at which alpha-adrenoceptor blockade influences decerebrate rigidity is not clear. Possible sites include:

(a) *The cerebellum*   It is highly likely that Purkinje cells in the cerebellum are inhibited by the noradrenergic pathways from the locus coeruleus (Siggins et al, 1973) but, since the Purkinje cells are themselves inhibitory to areas such as the lateral vestibular nucleus and cerebellar-subcortical nuclei (Eccles, 1966), blockade of their noradrenaline receptors would be likely to release tonic lateral vestibular drive and ongoing brain-stem activity.

(b) *The lateral vestibular nucleus*   Cells in this nucleus are consistently activated by iontophoretically applied noradrenaline (Yamamoto, 1967), as are a proportion of cells in the pontine and medullary reticular formation (Boakes et al, 1971). Noradrenergic pathways could themselves affect these cells but there is no supportive evidence that they do so.

(c) *Other brain-stem sites*

(d) *Spinal receptor sites*   Experiments in which brain-stem nuclei are stimulated electrically shed some light on the possible sites of action of drugs which influence adrenergic transmission. Alpha-adrenoceptor blockade appears to block the facilitatory influence of 8th cranial nerve stimulation on gastrocnemius muscle tension in the decerebrate cat (Barnes and Pompeiano, 1971). Grillner (1969) has reviewed recent research on the effects of stimulation of the lateral vestibular nucleus and a small area in the median longitudinal bundle on a- and γ-lumbar motoneurones. It is evident that neither of these pathways are likely to be noradrenergic since they are composed of large, fast conducting fibres while the catecholamine-containing axons are narrow and unmyelinated in the spinal cord. However, of considerable interest is the report by Grillner and Shik (1973) that stimulation of a region below the inferior colliculus induced loco-motion in precollicular, postmamillar cats by slow conducting pathways. They suggested that a noradrenergic locomotor reticulospinal system activated from a mesencephalic centre might be involved, but no further evidence has been published to support this suggestion.

Studies possibly relating alpha-adrenergic mechanisms and stretch reflex in man have been few. During the early clinical development of chlorpromazine its muscle relaxant effects in patient with spasticity were noted but its value on chronic dosing was disappointing. Matthews (1965) investigated the effect on spasticity of chlorproethazine, a drug with equal alpha-adrenoceptor blocking activity to that of chlorpromazine (Keary and Maxwell, 1967). Spastic hypertonus was reduced in 18 of 19 patients given chlorproethazine intravenously, but there was only minor relief of extensor spasms. EMG measures of tonic stretch reflex activity were reduced in both extensor and flexor lower limb muscles, the effects being most marked in patients with extensor spasticity and spinal lesions. H-reflexes were inhibited at the same time as tonic stretch reflexes, but to a less marked extent. On chronic therapy, however, the drug was relatively ineffective in treating spasticity, and adverse effects such as weakness and drowsiness were common.

Changes in H-reflex and triceps surae jerk amplitude in normal subjects after intravenous chlorpromazine and diazepam have recently been reported (Brunia, 1973). While both drugs reduced the jerk amplitude, the H-reflex was suppressed by diazepam only, suggesting that chlorpromazine's major effect is on fusimotor drive in man as in animals.

Studies in patients with Parkinson's disease (Andrews and Burke, 1973) and athetotic rigidity (Andrews, Neilson and Knowles, 1973) revealed stretch reflex changes after phenoxybenzamine administration compatible with those which would be expected if effects comparable to those of L-dopa in spinal animals were being blocked by the drug. The patients with Parkinson's disease were, in fact, receiving L-dopa, and the question arose as to how much its therapeutic action might be spinally mediated.

It is also of interest that in the 'stiff man syndrome' the degree of rigidity correlates with the urinary excretion of MHPG, the major cerebral metabolite of noradrenaline (Schmitt, Stahl and Spehlman, 1975) and that massive overdose of monoamine oxidase inhibitors produce rigidity in man (Robertson, 1972).

The work reported in this paper is a continuation of that started by Phillips, Richens and Shand (1973). As thymoxamine, probably the most specific alpha-adrenoceptor blocking drug available (Sugden, 1974), produced a marked reduction in the triceps surae jerk amplitude, it seemed logical to examine the possible therapeutic action of the drug in patients with spasticity. Phillips et al, (1973) had found that an intravenous infusion of noradrenaline sufficient to produce a marked pressor response was without effect on the tendon jerk response and concluded that the effect of thymoxamine (and methylamphetamine) was on the spinal cord rather than peripherally, e.g. on muscle spindles. Furthermore, as neither of the latter drugs modified H-reflex responses, they considered that the drugs were acting on the γ-efferent system, possibly by modifying transmission in a descending noradrenergic pathway which is facilitatory to fusimotor neurones supplying the gastrocnemius-soleus muscle (Figure 2).

Our first step was to verify in human volunteers the presence of a central alpha-adrenoceptor by studying the tendon jerk inhibiting potencies of compounds known to have alpha-adrenoceptor blocking properties. Having satisfied ourselves that a wide range of these drugs uniformly depressed tendon jerk responses, we proceeded to evaluate the most potent of these, thymoxamine, as an antispasticity agent in a small group of patients. This drug was compared with diazepam and with a placebo in a controlled trial, using the EMG response to muscle stretch as a measure of spasticity.

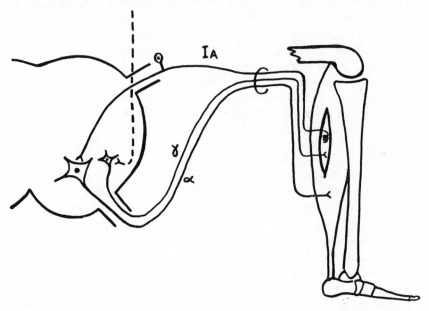

Figure 2   Diagram of the stretch reflex arc. The dashed line represents a possible noradrenergic pathway according to the suggestion of Phillips, Richens and Shand (1970).

SUBJECTS AND METHODS

Studies in volunteers

The tendon jerk inhibiting properties of seven drugs were compared with their ability to block pressor responses to infused noradrenaline in healthy volunteers, aged from 20 to 35 years.

The amplitude of the triceps surae jerk was measured isometrically using a modification of the method described by Phillips et al (1973). Full details have been given elsewhere (White, 1976). In brief, the subject lay on a bed with one leg raised over a padded Dexion frame. Mounted on the frame was a wooden footplate which was adjusted so that the foot was held slightly plantar flexed. The footplate was connected to a Grass FT 10C force-displacement transducer, with a maximum sensitivity range from 500 mg to 10 kg, which recorded iso-metric contraction of the triceps surae muscle. A weighted hammer was mounted on a pivot such that, on release, the projecting head hit the subject's Achilles tendon and and rebounded freely, eliciting the jerk. The hammer was dropped from a fixed height on each occasion. The output of the strain gauge was recorded on either a Devices M2 or a Mingograph recorder.

The tendon jerk was elicited ten times at random intervals of four to eight seconds. The amplitude of the trace was read with a ruler and the mean amplitude calculated for each set.

The peripheral alpha-adrenoceptor blocking potency of the antagonist drugs was assessed by determining their ability to block pressor responses to noradrenaline. The subjects were acclimatised in position for at least 15 minutes before starting. Blood pressure was then measured using a standard sphygmomanometer and the pulse rate taken by palpation of the radial artery. A set of control readings was taken and the blocking drug or placebo (saline) was then given as an injection over a two minute period into an antecubital fossa vein. Further readings of blood pressure, pulse rate and tendon jerk amplitude were obtained at 5, 10, and occasionally 15 minutes after the end of injection. The pressor responses to infusion of increasing doses of $(-)$ – noradrenaline tartrate (Levophed, Winthrop) $(8-60 \,\mu g/min)$ in 5% dextrose solution into an antecubital fossa vein were then measured. Five minutes were allowed for stabilisation at each level before blood pressure reading. Mean blood pressure (diastolic + ⅓ pulse pressure) was calculated. The infusion was continued until a mean blood pressure of 120 mmHg was reached.

The changes after the following seven drugs were compared with those after saline (0.9% NaCl w/v): Chlorpromazine hydrochloride (Largactil, May and Baker), 0.1 mg/kg; thioridazine hydrochloride (Melleril, Sandoz), 0.15 mg/kg; prochlorperazine mesylate (Stemetil, May and Baker), 0.1 mg/kg; dimethothiazine mesylate (Fusaban, May and Baker), 1.0 mg/kg; indoramin hydrochloride (John Wyeth and Bro.), 0.2 mg/kg; benzoctamine hydrochloride (Tacitin, Ciba), 0.2 mg/kg; and clonidine hydrochloride (Catapres, Boehringer Ingelheim), 2.0 μg/kg. Each of the drugs was given to six subjects except clonidine (N = 5), benzoctamine (N = 5) and indoramin (N = 11). They were administered on a randomised, double blind basis, using Latin squares for randomisation.

Studies in spastic patients

Changes in tonic and dynamic stretch reflex activity and grip strength in patients with spasticity were measured on three occasions, after intravenous injection of thymoxamine (0.1 mg/kg), diazepam (0.05 mg/kg) or placebo (saline).

Six patients were included, each having marked spastic hypertonia in one or both legs (Table I). The degree of spastic hypertonia was assessed using a specially designed apparatus on which the patient lay supine with his spastic leg raised over a frame and his foot held on to a flat wooden footpiece by straps (White, 1976). The footpiece was attached by a steel rod to one end of a hydraulic system driven by constant torque 1.5 horse power electric motor (Speedranger, J.H. Fenner & Co). The motor was controlled by limit switch system allowing virtually instantaneous stop and start, and could be operated manually or triggered automatically, in forward or reverse. The attachment of the rod to the footpiece was placed towards the ball of the foot so that during operation rotation of the foot took place about the ankle. The triceps surae muscle could therefore be passively stretched and relaxed. The degree of dorsiflexion or plantar flexion could be altered by adjustment of the apparatus, and an angular velocity of 10°/sec was chosen after several pilot studies. Silver-silver chloride skin EEG electrodes were placed approximately 8 cm apart over the soleus muscle for recording EMG activity. The EMG signal was fed into an integrator made in the Medical Electronics Department of St Bartholomew's Hospital. The integrator triggered the electric motor to produce a single movement of the foot. The EMG and other signals were recorded on an eight channel Mingograph EEG recorder. The total EMG activity was measured during five periods of dorsiflexion and five periods of plantar flexion of the foot at regular intervals, each integration period lasting 7 seconds from the start of the stretch. Baseline readings of EMG activity were made before and between readings during each session with the foot in a resting position, and a mean baseline reading for the session subtracted from each of the results.

TABLE I   Details of Patients with Spasticity

Subject	Age	Sex	Details of Lesion	Details of Disorder
1	32	M	Traumatic lesion of cord at 6th cervical segment 4 years previously.	Severe spastic quadriplegia, legs in extension, arms in partial flexion. Able to walk slowly with support.
2	53	M	Late onset disseminated sclerosis with plaque in high cervical region.	Mild weakness of arms. Marked rigid paraplegia. Able to walk slowly.
3	64	M	Cerebrovascular accident six months previously.	Severe right hemiplegia: arm in flexion, leg in extension.
4	19	M	Vertebral haemangioma: almost complete transverse cord lesion seen at operation, T9 level.	Severe spastic paraplegia. Both legs in flexed position. Frequent flexor spasms.
5	53	F	Longstanding disseminated sclerosis. Major lesion at T9 level.	Severe spastic paraplegia: legs in extension.
6	55	M	Longstanding, slowly progressive cervical lesion, probably disseminated sclerosis.	Marked quadriplegia. Spastic legs, in extension. Walked slowly.
7	61	M	Cerebrovascular accident three months previously.	Left hemiplegia. Absent tendon jerks in right leg.

Relative grip strength was determined using a dynamometer. For each set of readings the subject was asked to squeeze as hard as possible over five three second periods with three second intervals between them.

The procedure during each session was as follows: the subject lay in position on the couch for at least fifteen minutes before measurements were started. Two sets of control readings of mean blood pressure and pulse rate, EMG response in the soleus muscle, tendon jerk amplitude, and grip strength were taken, separated by five minutes. The intravenous injection was then given into an antecubital fossa vein over a one minute period. Further sets of readings were taken at 5, 10 and thirty minutes after the end of injection. Attempts were made to assess changes in tone clinically if an arm was affected by spasticity.

RESULTS

Studies in volunteers

The mean percentage changes in triceps surae jerk amplitude after each of the drugs together with group mean noradrenaline dose ratios are shown in Table II (more detailed results are given by White, 1976).

A reduction in tendon jerk amplitude was seen after administration of each of the blocking drugs, and this achieved statistical significance for chlorpromazine at five minutes after injection, and for chlorpromazine, dimethothiazine, benzoctamine, clonidine and indoramin at ten minutes after injection. Measurements with indoramin were continued to 15 minutes after injection when its peak effect appeared to have passed, and reduction in jerk amplitude was no longer significant.

TABLE II % changes (mean ± s.e. mean) in triceps surae jerk amplitude, and mean dose ratios of noradrenaline ± s.e. mean of changes in dose, after injection of each of the drugs. Results at equivalent times after placebo have been subtracted. N = 6, except where stated. Previously published results after injection of thymoxamine (Phillips et al, 1973) have been included for comparison.

| | Triceps surae jerk % changes | | | Noradrenaline |
	5 min	10 min	15 min	Dose Ratios
Dimethothiazine	-34 ± 13.4	-39 ± 11.7	–	1.40 ± 0.12
(1.0 mg/kg)	NS	$p < 0.02$		$p < 0.05$
Benzoctamine	-22 ± 9.3	-38 ± 7.2	–	1.71 ± 0.22
(0.2 mg/kg)	NS	$p < 0.01$		$p < 0.05$
Chlorpromazine	-29 ± 5.4	-37 ± 3.7	–	1.96 ± 0.32
(0.1 mg/kg)	$p < 0.01$	$p < 0.01$		$p < 0.05$
Clonidine	-28 ± 12.5	-23 ± 7.5	–	see text
(2.0 μg/kg)	NS	$p < 0.05$		
Indoramin	-15 ± 6.4	-22 ± 7.7	-12 ± 6.1	1.92 ± 0.18
(0.2 mg/kg)	NS	$p < 0.05$	NS	$p < 0.01$
	(n = 11)	(n = 6)	(n = 11)	
Prochlorperazine	-40 ± 18.2	-18 ± 8.2	–	1.13 ± 0.16
(0.1 mg/kg)	NS	NS		NS
Thioridazine	-3 ± 2.6	-10 ± 4.9	–	1.51 ± 0.14
(0.15 mg/kg)	NS	NS		$p < 0.02$
Thymoxamine	-62 ± 5.0			
(0.1 mg/kg)	$p < 0.005$			
Thymoxamine	-71 ± 6.5			
(0.2 mg/kg)	$p < 0.001$			

Significant displacement to the right of noradrenaline pressor dose-response curves was found following each of the drugs except prochlorperazine and clonidine. The parallelism of the dose-response curves was felt to be satisfactory on visual inspection except on one occasion after clonodine, though statistical analysis for parallelism was not applied. A plateau in response to increasing doses of noradrenaline was sometimes seen with relatively modest rises in blood pressure after active drugs. This was attributed to unmasking of the beta-agonist action of the larger doses of noradrenaline used during alpha-adrenoceptor blockade.

Injection of clonidine was followed by reduction in tendon jerk amplitude in all subjects. Changes in sensitivity to noradrenaline after this drug were variable, however, with individual dose ratios, where calculable, of 0.61, 1.52, 1.61 and 5.12. In the other subject, inhibition of pressor responses occurred but the disparities in the dose-response curves prevented quantitation.

Assessment of the changes following prochlorperazine was complicated by the occurrence of marked and distressing restlessness in two subjects, presumably acute akathisia which made their tendon jerk responses variable and difficult to assess.

Sedation was seen after each of the drugs except thioridazine. It was particularly marked after chlorpromazine, dimethothiazine and indoramin, though no subject ever became unrousable. Some subjects appeared to sleep through the experiment after indoramin without change in jerk size from control readings. Thioridazine produced no detectable central nervous side effects.

In the period after injection and before noradrenaline infusion, a significant increase in resting pulse rate occurred after only chlorpromazine. One subject not included in the series developed syncope about 5 minutes after chlorpromazine injection when in the chair with undetectable pulse and blood pressure, which was rapidly reversed by laying him flat. Otherwise no consistent or significant changes occurred in resting pulse rate or blood pressure before NA infusion after any of the drugs.

It was apparent on visual inspection that little correlation existed between pressor response blockade and tendon jerk changes after the drugs. The results due to clonidine were excluded from correlation analysis. Neither group mean nor individual change analyses showed significance: $r = -0.21$ and 0.01 respectively.

Studies in patients

Individual changes in integrated EMG activity and triceps surae jerk amplitude are shown in Tables III and IV.

Injection of thymoxamine was followed by significant reductions in EMG activity in the soleus muscle in response to both stretch and shortening, at 5, 10 and 30 minutes after injection. The duration of EMG response reduction exceeded that of sedation and facial flushing due to the drug, and maximum change was at 30 minutes whereas the sedation was maximal at 2–5 minutes.

The EMG response to soleus muscle movement was also reduced after diazepam, but less consistently. The changes were less marked than those after thymoxamine, but there was no significant difference between the group mean changes. Diazepam's effect on integrated EMG also persisted beyond the period of sedation.

134

TABLE III Percentage changes in EMG response to muscle stretch in six spastic patients

Subject	5 min after Thymoxamine 0.1 mg/kg	5 min after Diazepam 0.05 mg/kg	5 min after N. Saline
1	−100	−50	+ 22
2	− 85	−49	+ 25
3	− 69	−75	+ 43
4	+ 25	−39	− 13
5	− 81	−54	− 40
6	− 60	+ 5	− 9

TABLE IV Mean % changes (± s.e. mean) in triceps surae jerk amplitude after injection of thymoxamine and diazepam

After thymoxamine 0.1 mg/kg
5 min	−25	± 7	$p < 0.02$
10 min	−13	±10	N.S.
30 min	−26	± 4	$p < 0.01$

After diazepam 0.05 mg/kg
5 min	−15	± 6	N.S.
10 min	0	± 7	N.S.
30 min	− 2	± 6	N.S.

After injection of both thymoxamine and diazepam, the EMG reaction to muscle shortening was reduced as well as the response to stretch. The clonus present in subject 4 was abolished by diazepam and reduced by thymoxamine. EMG activity both while the foot was being moved and while it was held in dorsiflexion was reduced by both drugs in all subjects.

Mean reductions of tendon jerk amplitude were statistically significant at 5 and 30 minutes after thymoxamine, but not at other times. Subject 4, with an almost complete cord lesion, showed little reduction in jerk size after either drug.

Changes in grip strength were not consistent, and there was no evidence of induced weakness in most of the subjects. The two hemiplegic patients, however, both complained of marked weakness in the affected arm after thymoxamine and this was seen as 91 and 85% reductions in grip strength. No such complaint occurred after diazepam.

No significant changes were seen in blood pressure or pulse rate except a small increase in the latter at thirty minutes after thymoxamine. Diazepam tended to produce larger decreases in blood pressure and pulse rate than thymoxamine.

Two subjects were given thymoxamine openly while ambulant: subjects 1 and 6. Both patients were given increasing intravenous doses at ten minute intervals to a total of 0.16 mg/kg, while tone in arms and legs, power and walking speed were assessed clinically. Facial flushing and slight drowsiness were seen in both patients for a short period after the higher doses, and a small fall in blood pressure was seen in subject 6 who was also transiently euphoric. There appear to be small reductions in hypertonicity in both patients' legs and in the arms of subject 1 but the changes were not striking.

One further patient was given intravenous thymoxamine at a dose of 10mg. Aged 19, he was severely demented with bilateral decerebrate rigidity. He showed no response to thymoxamine at that dose.

DISCUSSION

Studies in volunteers

These experiments were designed to test the hypothesis that central noradrenergic pathways facilitate muscle stretch reflexes in man by (i) determining whether all drugs with alpha-adrenoceptor blocking activity reduced tendon jerk reflexes, and (ii) by comparing the degree of depression of the tendon jerk with the degree of blockade of alpha-adrenoceptor mechanisms in the cardiovascular system.

Although the first objective was achieved, and the results supported the hypothesis, the lack of correlation between the central and peripheral effects of the blocking drugs was disappointing. Some drugs, e.g. chlorpromazine, produced a much greater reversal of noradrenaline pressor effects than others, e.g. dimethothiazine, despite their causing a similar degree of reduction of the triceps surae jerk (TSJ).

The results suggest that thymoxamine is consistently more potent than other drugs as a TSJ depressant, and two to three times as potent in this respect as indoramin. Thymoxamine's duration of action in man is too short for adequate assessment of peripheral a-adrenoceptor blockade, but it has been consistently reported as a weaker a-adrenoceptor blocker than chlorpromazine or indoramin in vitro (Sugden, 1974).

The lack of correlation of either pressor response or TSJ inhibition with degrees of sedation is also striking. Indoramin produced relatively slight tendon jerk change with marked sedation. Thioridazine considerably inhibited NA pressor responses without sedation.

The failure to demonstrate a correlation between peripheral and central effects of the alpha-adrenoceptor blocking drugs may have been due to a number of factors. In order to exert a central action the drugs have to enter the central nervous system and achieve an adequate concentration at central receptor sites. For a good correlation to be seen between peripheral and central effects the concentrations at both sites would have to be similar. It is likely that pharmacokinetic differences between the various compounds used in this study, e.g. the rate at which they penetrate the blood-brain barrier, would have produced widely differing concentration ratios.

It is possible that pharmacological effects other than alpha-adrenoceptor blockade could have been responsible for the reduction in tendon jerk responses, as it is known that most of the blocking drugs used have other actions, such as 5–HT and cholinergic receptor blockade. The lack of correlation between the sedative and tendon jerk effects of this series of drugs supports such a suggestion.

Finally, it should be noted that, for practical reasons, all the blocking drugs could not be tested in the same subjects. This produces the difficulty that comparison between drugs also, to some extent, involves a comparison between subjects, and this is methodologically unsatisfactory.

Studies in patients

During dorsiflexion of the foot in the apparatus used, stretching of the triceps surae muscle occurred but at the same time considerable pressure was exerted on the sole of the foot, which is an area in which noxious stimulation induces generalised flexion responses in spastic legs (Dimitrijevic and Nathan, 1968; Kungelberg et al, 1960). During plantar flexion not only was the triceps surae muscle being shortened and antagonists stretched but pressure was put on the dorsum of the foot as it was pulled down by straps. It is evident that a variety of stimuli were likely to be generating afferent impulses. Primary and secondary muscle spindle endings, Golgi tendon organs and cutaneous receptors, particularly for pressure, were probably activated.

Responses to muscle shortening have been noted by a variety of workers, including Rushworth (1961) and Andrews, Burke and Lance (1972) who observed a shortening reaction in normal subjects during reinforcement as well as in spastic and Parkinsonian patients. Three normal subjects were tested on the present apparatus and no triceps surae EMG responses could be detected during relaxation. The findings of Andrews, Burke and Lance (1972) confirm those of Rushworth (1961) and Denny-Brown (1960) in that the static element of the shortening reaction is likely to be due to activation of stretch receptors in the antagonist muscle, since infiltration of the antagonist with procaine abolished the response, but the same does not apparently apply to the shortening reaction during movement, which is autogenic. A complication in the present experiments was that as the series of ten movements progressed, EMG activity tended to become continuous, and an exaggeration of EMG responses occurred presumably as a response to total afferent activation. We agree with Dimitrijevic and Nathan's hypothesis (1967a, 1967b) that spasticity is in large part, in patients with spinal lesions at least, a state of hyper-responsiveness to all afferent neuronal activity owing to the loss of supraspinal inhibitory influences. The disinhibited reflex

137

responses to all stimulation in these experiments would therefore appear to be a good measure of spasticity, and probably the best measure is that with combined dorsiflexion and plantar flexion EMG readings.

The population tested in this study, though limited in number, was heterogeneous in terms of location of their CNS lesions. Subject 4 had a nearly complete cord lesion at the T9 level, whereas subjects 3 and 7 were hemiplegic after cerebrovascular accidents. The remainder had partial spinal lesions. No change in EMG responses were seen at five minutes after injection of thymoxamine in subject 4, though EMG activity was reduced at ten and thirty minutes. The amount of clonus on dorsiflexion of his foot was reduced, as was an apparent crossed flexor response seen by depression of the contralateral footplate during dorsiflexion.

The reduction in triceps surae jerk amplitude was by no means as marked as has been seen in normal subjects. In only one subject (3) was measurement made on a leg unaffected by spasticity, and it seems possible that the loss of descending pathways may have produced a disturbed balance of supraspinal influences and a reduced response to thymoxamine.

The striking weakness seen in the two hemiplegic subjects could be due to a similar action of thymoxamine to that seen in the decerebrate animal. Movements in these subjects are presumably imposed on tonic muscle contraction due to released supraspinal drive, and abolition of that would be likely to cause apparent weakness. Weakness has been observed in studies both on diazepam (Nathan, 1970) and chlorproethazine (Matthews, 1965), though not only in patients with high supraspinal lesions.

It seems reasonable to conclude from this study that thymoxamine can markedly inhibit spastic hyper-reactivity in a variety of patients after intravenous dosing. There are some suggestions from the evidence that its effect may depend on the presence of supraspinal influences although it is not possible to say at what level in the central nervous system the drug is producing its effect.

The original hypothesis of Phillips et al (1973) that blockade of a descending noradrenergic influence on fusimotor neurones was responsible for the reduction in spinal reflex activity is probably no longer tenable because, in the resting state, there is little activity in Ia afferents in normal subjects (D. Burke, personal communication) and therefore a further relaxation of the muscle spindle would not account for the marked reduction in tendon jerks produced by thymoxamine. The effect of this drug may, however, be on noradrenergic pathways which are involved at some other point in the overall control of spinal reflex activity.

The benefit which thymoxamine appeared to confer on the patients in this study suggested that a trial of the drug administered orally would be worthwhile. Unfortunately, however, it is poorly and unreliably absorbed by this route and therefore it was not considered practical to pursue this line of research. The development of a well-absorbed alpha-adrenergic blocker as specific as thymoxamine would be invaluable.

Acknowledgements

We would like to thank Action for the Crippled Child, the Central Research Fund of the University of London, William Warner and Co. Ltd, and John Wyeth and Brother Ltd for financial assistance.

References

Anden, N-E, Butcher, S G, Corrodi, M, Fuxe, K and Ungerstedt, U (1970) *European Journal of Pharmacology, 11, 303*
Anden, N-E, Carlsson, A, Hillarp, N-Å and Magnusson, T (1965) *Life of Science, 4,* 129
Anden, N-E and Fuxe, K E (1971) *British Journal of Pharmacology, 43,* 747
Anden, N-E, Haggendal, J, Magnusson, T and Rosengren, E (1964) *Acta physiologica scandinavica, 62,* 115
Anden, N-E, Jukes, M G M, Lundberg, A and Vyklicky, L (1966a) *Acta physiologica scandinavica, 67,* 373
Anden, N-E, Jukes, M G M, Lundberg, A and Vyklicky, L (1966a) *Acta physiologica scandinavica, 68,* 322
Andrews, C J and Burke, D (1973) *Journal of Neurology, Neurosurgery and Psychiatry, 36,* 328
Andrews, C J, Burke, D and Lance, J W (1972) *Brain, 95,* 795
Andrews, C J, Neilson, P and Knowles, L (1973) *Journal of Neurology, Neurosurgery and Psychiatry, 36,* 94
Barnes, C D and Pompeiano, O (1971) *Neuropharmacology, 10,* 425
Boakes, R J, Bradley, P B, Brookes, N, Candy, J M and Wolstencroft, J H (1971) *British Journal of Pharmacology, 41,* 462
Brunia, C H M (1973) In: *New Developments in Electromyography and Clinical Neurophysiology.* Ed: J E Desmedt, S Karger, Basle. Pages 367–370.
Dahlstrom, A and Fuxe, K (1965) *Acta physiologica scandinavica, 64, suppl. 247,* 1
Denny-Brown, D (1960) *Lancet, ii,* 1099
Denny-Brown, D (1966) *The Cerebral Control of Movement, Sherrington Lectures, No.8.* University Press, Liverpool
Dhawan, B N and Sharma, J N (1970) *British Journal of Pharmacology, 40,* 237
Dimitrievic, M R and Nathan, P W (1967a) *Brain, 90,* 1
Dimitrievic, M R and Nathan, P W (1967b) *Brain, 90,* 333
Dimitrievic, M R and Nathan, P W (1968) *Brain, 90,* 349
Eccles, J C (1966) *Muscle Afferents and Motor Control* Ed: R Granit, Stockholm, Almquist and Wiksell. Pages 19–36
Ellaway, P H and Pascoe, J E (1968) *Journal of Physiology, 197,* 8
Fedina, L, Lundberg, A and Vysklicky, L (1971) *Acta physiologica scandinavica, 83,* 495
Grillner, S (1969) *Acta physiologica scandinavica, Suppl. 327*
Grillner, S and Shik, M L (1973) *Acta physiologica scandinavica, 87,* 320
Janssen, P A J (1970) *Modern Problems in Pharmacopsychiatry. Vol. 5.*
    Eds: F A Freyhan, N. Petrilowitsch, P Pichot, S Karger, Basle. Pages 33–43
Keary, E M and Maxwell, D R (1967) *British Journal of Pharmacology, 29,* 400
Kungelberg, E, Eklund, E and Grimby, L (1960) *Brain, 83,* 394
Martin, W R and Eades, C G (1967) *Psychopharmacology, 11,* 195

Matthews, W B (1965) *Brain, 88,* 1057

Maxwell, D R, Read, M A and Sumpter, E A (1974) *British Journal of Pharmacology, 50,* 35

Maxwell, D R and Sumpter, E A (1972) *Journal of Physiology, 222,* 173

Nathan, P W (1970) *Journal of Neurological Science, 10,* 33

Phillips, S, Richens, A and Shand, D G (1973) *British Journal of Pharmacology, 47,* 595

Robertson, J C (1972) *Postgraduate Medical Journal, 48,* 64

Rushworth, G (1960) *Journal of Neurology, Neurosurgery and Psychiatry, 23,* 99

Schmidt, R T, Stahl, S M and Spehlmann, R (1975) *Neurology, 25,* 622

Siggins, G R, Battenberg, E F, Hoffer, B J and Bloom, F E (1973) *Science, 179,* 585

Sugden, R F (1974) *British Journal of Pharmacology, 51,* 467

White, C de Bois (1976) *MD Thesis. University of London. Pharmacological studies of spinal and cardiovascular α-adrenergic mechanisms in man.*

Yamamoto, C (1967) *Journal of Pharmacology and Experimental Therapeutics, 156,* 39

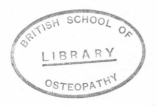

INDEX

A

Abiotrophy, 30–4, 68, 70, 122
Acrylamide neuropathy, 45
Aetiolology (*see* Motor Neurone Disease)
Ageusia, 9
Age incidence in motor neurone disease (*see* Motor Neurone Disease)
Alcohol, 6
Alpha-adrenoceptor blocking agents, 125–38
Alzheimer's disease, 3, 102, 110
Amyotrophic lateral sclerosis (ALS), 1, 2, 4, 62, 64, 66, 78, 79, 81, 103, 121
 aetiology of, 17, 22, 26, 27
 definition of, 15, 18
 epidemiology of, 14–27
 fasciculation in, 4, 15, 103
 incidence of, 15
 sporadic form of, 26, 27, 74, 103
 treatment of, 26
American Association of Neuropathologists, 102
Ankle clonus, 4
Anoxia, 68
Anterior horn cells, 1, 7, 15, 32, 42, 64, 99
 abnormalities in, 15; in ALS, 18, 46
 changes in, 65, 76, 95, 122
 degeneration of, 19, 32, 67, 94, 107
 in hereditary neuropathies, 53–8
Aran, 1
Ataxia, 103
Atrophies
 chronic, 4
 groups of, 9, 55, 56, 66, 82, 86, 114
 hereditary, 55
 muscular, 1, 2, 3, 15, 18, 92
 spinal muscular, 53, 54, 112–19
Awjn tribe, the, 3
Axonal neuropathies, 44, 77
Axonal transport, 36–49

B

Babinski, 4
Bell, Sir Charles, 1
Beri-beri, 77
Bilabial plosives ('p and b'), 5
Biopsies, studies of, 9, 49, 79–93
   muscle, 12
Bulbar palsy, 1, 2, 3, 4–12, 80
   aetiology of, 8, 121
   associations, 7
   chronic, 2, 92
   diagnosis of, 9, 121
   progressive, 4
   presentation of, 5
   pseudo-, 2, 4, 5, 6, 15

C

Cancer, 23, 46
Caroline Islands, incidence of motor neurone disease in, 17
Carrell, Alexis, 31
Carrier molecule theory, the, 41, 42
'Cell death, physiological', 31, 32, 33, 34, 64, 75, 76, 77, 123
Cell structure, 36, 76
Cerebral arteriosclerosis, 8
Cerebrovascular disease, 4
Cervical spondylosis, 8
Charcot, 1
Charcot-Marie-Tooth disease, 49
Charing Cross Hospital, research at, 80
'Chequerboard pattern', the, 80, 84, 85, 86, 87, 89, 80
Chomorro tribe, incidence of motor neurone disease in the, 3
Circulatory disturbance, 68
Clark's column, 75, 103, 104, 106
'Claw hand', 3
Compression, 4
Conduction velocities, 15
Creutzfeldt-Jakob disease (CJD), 123
Cruveilhier, 1
Cumulative Index Medicus, 31
Cycad, the, 25, 27
   Conference (1972), 24
Cycadin, 3
Cytoplasmic movement, 40
Cyton, the, 37–8, 42, 45
   protein synthesis in, 48

D

Davidenjow's syndrome, 56

Death (*see* Motor Neurone Disease)
Denervation in motor neurone disease, 9, 15, 91, 92, 95, 114
Demyelination, 19
Diagnosis (*see* Motor Neurone Disease)
Duchenne, 1
    muscular dystrophy, 118
Dysarthria, 5, 6, 62
Dysphagia, 6, 82
Dysphonia, 5
Dyspnoea, 5

E

Electromyography (EMG), 9, 11, 12, 81, 109, 123
    data in spinal muscular atrophy, 112–19, 138
Emotional lability, 4, 5
Encephalitis lethargica, 64, 68, 102, 121
Eosinophilic inclusions, 3
Epidemiology (*see* Motor Neurone Disease)

F

Familial form (*see* Motor Neurone Disease)
Fasciculation, 2, 4, 9, 11, 12, 57, 58, 65, 68, 95, 103
    benign, 9
    chronic, 4
    in ALS, 4, 15, 103
    of the tongue, 8, 9, 10
Fatiguability, 4
Fibre grouping, 82, 92, 93
Fibrillation changes, 9, 12, 17, 19, 64, 82
    Alzheimer, 3, 102, 110
Filippinos, incidence of motor neurone disease in, 3, 17
'Floppy baby', the, 10, 11
Foot drop, 8
Friedrich's ataxia, 74

G

Gamma globulin, 9
ganglia, 74, 76
Gastrectomy, 65, 67
Gastronomy, 9, 65
Gene mutation research in, 33
Geographical incidence (*see* Motor Neurone Disease)
Gliosis, 73, 75, 107
Glosso-labio-laryngeal paralysis, 1
Gower's sign, 12, 30

143

Greenfield's Neuropathology, 62
Guam, study of motor neurone disease in, 3, 17, 19, 24, 110

H

Hammersmith Hospital, research at, 65
Handbook of Clinical Neurology, 60
Hawaii, study of motor neurone disease in, 3, 17
Hayflick's phase, 32, 111
Hyperreflexia, 4
Hyperrhinolalia, 5
Hypertonia, 4
Hypoglycaemia, 65
Huntington's chorea, 7

I

Immunological studies, 23
'Infantile paralysis' (*see* Poliomyelitis)
International Classification of Diseases, 15

J

Jakob's disease, 64, 123
Japan, incidence of motor neurone disease in, 3, 16
Jaquai, study of motor neurone disease in, 3
Jaw jerks, 4

K

Kii Peninsular, study of motor neurone disease in, 3, 16, 19
Kugelberg-Welander syndrome (proximal MA), 10, 11, 112, 113, 115, 116

L

Lathyrus fruit, 3
Laryngeal palsy, 5
Ligation experiments, 37
Lower Motor Neurone disease (*see* Motor Neurone Disease)
Luys, 1

M

Macroglobulinaemia, 67, 68
'Main de singe', 3
Mariana Islands, the, 3, 16, 17, 20

Papua, study of Motor Neurone Disease in, 3
Parkinsonism-dementia (PD), 3, 5, 6, 7, 17, 64, 66, 110, 122, 137
Pathological laughter, 5
Percussion, 4
Perikaryon, 107
Pharyngeal stasis, 6
Pick's dementia, 7, 110
Poliomyelitis, paralytic, 63, 122
Polymositis, 9
Polyneuritis, 8
Primary lateral sclerosis, 15
Progressive dementia, 17
Progressive muscular atrophy (PMA), 1, 2, 3, 9, 10, 15, 81
   death from, 16
   fasciculation in, 4, 9
   following poliomyelitis, 63
   spinal, 53
Progressive vacuolar degeneration, 44
Prostigmine, 9
Protein (CSF), 9, 36, 97, 101
   species in axonal transport, 39, 47
   synthetic machinery, 48
Pseudobulbar palsy (*see* Bulbar palsy)
Ptosis, 11
Pulse-labelling experiments, 37–8
Purkinje cells, 128

R

Race incidence (*see* Motor Neurone Disease)
Radio-therapy, 9
Reflux oesophagitis, 6
Re-innervation in Motor Neurone Disease, 9, 89, 90, 92, 93
Retrograde transport, 40, 43
Riley-Day syndrome, 56
Roussy-Lévy syndrome, 56
Royal Free Hospital, research at the, 57

S

Salivation, 5, 9
Scapuloperoneal syndrome, 55, 56
Schwann cells, 40, 43, 45, 48
Sex incidence (*see* Motor Neurone Disease)
Semon's Law, 5
Sensory loss, 55
Spastic paraplegia, 7, 8 (*see also* Spasticity)
Spasticity, 4, 5, 62, 125–38
   familial, 7, 56
   symptoms of, 132

Speech, 5, 6, 10, 95
Spinal meningovascular syphilis, 64
Spinal muscular atrophy (*see* Atrophies)
Stabilising neurotubules, 39
Staining patterns, 75, 79, 80, 122
'Stiff man syndrome', 129
Strychnine, use of, 9
Supranuclear innervation, 2
Surae jerk, 130, 133, 137, 138
Swallowing, 6, 9, 10, 95
Symptoms (*see* Motor Neurone Disease)

T

Target fibres, 87
Thenar eminence, 3, 7
Thiamine deficiency, 77
Thyrotoxic myopathy, 9
Tongue, atrophy of the, 4, 5, 8, 10
Touch, 4
Tracheostomy, 9
Transport mechanisms, 33, 36–49, 75, 80, 128
Transport filament theory, 41
Treatment (*see* Motor Neurone Disease)
Triceps jerk, 3, 130, 138

U

Upper motor neurone disease (*see* Motor Neurone Disease)

V

Vincristine neuropathies, 45
Virus infection, 25, 64
    slow, 121–3
Vulpian-Bernardt syndrome, 3

W

Wallerian degeneration, 37
Wasting, 3, 7, 66, 81, 95, 96
Werdnig-Hoffman syndrome (Infantile MA), 10, 11, 53, 74
Werner's syndrome, 32

X

Xeroderma pigmentosum, 33
Xerostomia, 9
X-ray, 7